# Orthopaedics

pocket tutor

# Orthopaedics

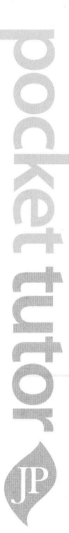

**Nicola Blucher** BA (Hons) MBBS MRCS (Eng)
Specialist Registrar in Trauma and Orthopaedics
North West Thames, London Deanery
London, UK

**Katherine Butler** BSc (Hons) MBBCh MRCS (Eng)
Core Trainee in Trauma and Orthopaedics
Royal Berkshire NHS Foundation Trust
Reading, UK

**Simon Platt** MB ChB FRCS (T&O) PGCert
Consultant Trauma and Orthopaedic Surgeon
Gold Coast University Hospital
Honorary Adjunct Associate Professor
Bond University
Queensland, Australia

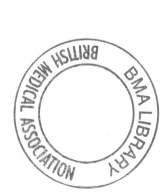

JP
medical
publishers

© 2017 JP Medical Ltd.

Published by JP Medical Ltd, 83 Victoria Street, London, SW1H 0HW, UK

Tel: +44 (0)20 3170 8910          Fax: +44 (0)20 3008 6180

Email: info@jpmedpub.com          Web: www.jpmedpub.com

**ISBN: 978-1-907816-99-4**

**British Library Cataloguing in Publication Data**
A catalogue record for this book is available from the British Library

**Library of Congress Cataloging in Publication Data**
A catalog record for this book is available from the Library of Congress

| Publisher: | Richard Furn |
| Development Editors: | Thomas Fletcher, Paul Mayhew |
| Editorial Assistants: | Katie Pattullo, Adam Rajah |
| Design: | Designers Collective Ltd |

# Preface

All doctors come into contact with patients who have musculo-skeletal disorders; *Pocket Tutor Orthopaedics* is a comprehensive, concise and clear guide to this specialty.

Chapters 1 and 2 open the book by covering the principles of orthopaedic examination, investigations and management. Subsequently, each chapter covers the conditions of a specific region, describing clinical features, relevant imaging modalities and options for definitive treatment. Throughout, the text is enriched with supportive diagrams and pertinent radiographs.

This book enables rapid access to topics in orthopaedics, which makes it invaluable to medical students as well as junior doctors working in orthopaedics or the emergency department.

We hope that you will find *Pocket Tutor Orthopaedics* useful on the ward, in clinic, in theatre, in the emergency department and in achieving examination success.

**Nicola Blucher, Katherine Butler, Simon Platt**
February 2017

# Contents

*Preface*                                           *v*
*Dedications and acknowledgements*                 *xi*

## Chapter 1  General principles
1.1    Fractures and dislocations                   1
1.2    Consent                                       6

## Chapter 2  Clinical essentials
2.1    Common symptoms and how to take a history    11
2.2    Clinical signs and examination               21
2.3    Investigations                               37
2.4    Management                                   45

## Chapter 3  Spine
3.1    Clinical scenario                            55
3.2    Anatomy                                      56
3.3    Examination                                  63
3.4    Cauda equina syndrome                        67
3.5    Spinal fractures                             70
3.6    Spinal cord injury                           78
3.7    Spinal metastases                            80
3.8    Other conditions                             83

## Chapter 4  Shoulder
4.1    Clinical scenario                            85
4.2    Anatomy                                      87
4.3    Examination                                  96
4.4    Clavicular fractures                         97
4.5    Acromioclavicular joint injuries            102
4.6    Scapular fractures                          104
4.7    Shoulder dislocations                       106
4.8    Rotator cuff injuries                       111
4.9    Proximal humeral fractures                  114
4.10   Humeral shaft fractures                     118
4.11   Brachial plexus injuries                    121
4.12   Biceps tendon injuries                      123

## Chapter 5  Elbow

| | | |
|---|---|---|
| 5.1 | Clinical scenario | 125 |
| 5.2 | Anatomy | 127 |
| 5.3 | Examination | 128 |
| 5.4 | Elbow dislocation | 131 |
| 5.5 | Supracondylar fractures (distal humeral fractures) | 134 |
| 5.6 | Olecranon fractures | 137 |
| 5.7 | Capitellum fractures | 139 |
| 5.8 | Radial head and neck fractures | 141 |
| 5.9 | Other conditions | 144 |

## Chapter 6  Wrist and hand

| | | |
|---|---|---|
| 6.1 | Clinical scenario | 147 |
| 6.2 | Anatomy | 148 |
| 6.3 | Examination | 151 |
| 6.4 | Mid-shaft fractures of the forearm | 153 |
| 6.5 | Distal radius fractures | 156 |
| 6.6 | Distal radioulnar joint injuries | 160 |
| 6.7 | Scaphoid fractures | 162 |
| 6.8 | Lunate and perilunate dislocations | 166 |
| 6.9 | Metacarpal fractures | 170 |
| 6.10 | Phalangeal fractures | 173 |
| 6.11 | Base-of-thumb fractures | 176 |
| 6.12 | Tendon (flexor and extensor) injuries of the wrist and hand | 178 |
| 6.13 | Flexor tendon sheath infection | 182 |
| 6.14 | Nail bed injuries | 183 |
| 6.15 | Paronychia | 185 |
| 6.16 | Other carpal fractures | 185 |

## Chapter 7  Hip

| | | |
|---|---|---|
| 7.1 | Clinical scenario | 187 |
| 7.2 | Anatomy | 188 |
| 7.3 | Examination | 190 |
| 7.4 | Hip dislocation | 193 |
| 7.5 | Neck of femur fractures | 197 |
| 7.6 | Femoral shaft fractures | 209 |
| 7.7 | Periprosthetic hip fractures | 212 |
| 7.8 | Osteoarthritis | 214 |

| 7.9 | Paget's disease of bone | 217 |
| 7.10 | Other conditions | 218 |

**Chapter 8  Pelvis**
| 8.1 | Clinical scenario | 221 |
| 8.2 | Anatomy | 222 |
| 8.3 | Examination | 225 |
| 8.4 | Pelvic fractures | 226 |
| 8.5 | Acetabular fractures | 232 |
| 8.6 | Sacral fractures | 236 |
| 8.7 | Coccygeal fractures | 238 |

**Chapter 9  Knee**
| 9.1 | Clinical scenario | 239 |
| 9.2 | Anatomy | 240 |
| 9.3 | Examination | 246 |
| 9.4 | Patellar fractures | 248 |
| 9.5 | Patellar dislocation | 252 |
| 9.6 | Tibial plateau fractures | 253 |
| 9.7 | Tibial shaft fractures | 257 |
| 9.8 | Distal femoral fractures | 259 |
| 9.9 | Quadriceps and patellar tendon injuries | 261 |
| 9.10 | Soft tissue injuries | 263 |
| 9.11 | Osteoarthritis | 265 |
| 9.12 | Knee dislocation | 267 |

**Chapter 10  Foot and ankle**
| 10.1 | Clinical scenario | 271 |
| 10.2 | Anatomy | 272 |
| 10.3 | Examination | 274 |
| 10.4 | Ankle fractures | 279 |
| 10.5 | Pilon fractures | 285 |
| 10.6 | Ankle sprains | 289 |
| 10.7 | Talus fractures | 291 |
| 10.8 | Calcaneal fractures | 294 |
| 10.9 | Achilles tendon ruptures | 297 |
| 10.10 | Lisfranc (tarsometatarsal) injuries | 300 |
| 10.11 | Metatarsal fractures | 303 |
| 10.12 | Phalangeal fractures | 308 |
| 10.13 | Other conditions | 310 |

## Chapter 11  Paediatric orthopaedics

| | | |
|---|---|---|
| 11.1 | Clinical scenario | 313 |
| 11.2 | Examination | 315 |
| 11.3 | Growth plate fractures | 315 |
| 11.4 | Supracondylar humeral fractures | 319 |
| 11.5 | Condylar fractures | 322 |
| 11.6 | Radial head and neck fractures | 327 |
| 11.7 | Radial head subluxation | 329 |
| 11.8 | Hip problems: slipped upper femoral epiphysis | 330 |
| 11.9 | Hip problems: Perthes' disease | 333 |
| 11.10 | Hip problems: transient synovitis | 334 |
| 11.11 | Femoral shaft fractures | 335 |
| 11.12 | Tibial fractures | 338 |
| 11.13 | Non-accidental injuries | 339 |
| 11.14 | Osteogenesis imperfecta | 341 |

## Chapter 12  Orthopaedic trauma

| | | |
|---|---|---|
| 12.1 | Clinical scenario | 343 |
| 12.2 | Advanced Trauma Life Support | 345 |
| 12.3 | Open fractures | 346 |
| 12.4 | Compartment syndrome | 349 |
| 12.5 | Vascular injuries | 352 |

## Chapter 13  Orthopaedic infections and other soft tissue problems

| | | |
|---|---|---|
| 13.1 | Clinical scenario | 355 |
| 13.2 | Septic arthritis | 356 |
| 13.3 | Osteomyelitis | 358 |
| 13.4 | Gangrene | 360 |
| 13.5 | Necrotising fasciitis | 362 |
| 13.6 | Postoperative wound infections | 363 |
| 13.7 | Cellulitis | 364 |
| 13.8 | Abscesses | 365 |
| 13.9 | Foot ulcers | 367 |
| 13.10 | Foreign bodies | 369 |
| 13.11 | Bite injuries | 371 |
| 13.12 | Neuropathic arthropathy | 372 |

| | |
|---|---|
| *Index* | *375* |

# Dedications and acknowledgements

Thanks to Paul Evans, Gillian Jackson, Jeremy Kaye, Gunasekaran Kumar, Ashok Lal Ramavath, Roger Walton and Hafiz Yakob for their help sourcing images.

**NB, KB, SP**

For Catherine, David Blucher and Andrew Blucher.

**NB**

For my parents.

**SP**

Figures 3.6–7, 4.7, 4.9–11. 4.22, 5.1–3, 6.2, 6.4, 7.1a, 7.4–6, 8.1–2, 9.1–3, 10.1–2 and 10.4–5 are copyright of Sam Scott-Hunter and are reproduced from: Tunstall R, Shah N. Pocket Tutor Surface Anatomy. London: JP Medical Publishers, 2012.

Figures 2.3, 3.8, 4.12, 5.4, 6.5–8, 9.7, 10.6–7, are reproduced from: Cartledge P, Cartledge K, Lockey A. Pocket Tutor Clinical Examination. London: JP Medical Publishers, 2012.

Figures 2.4 a and b are reproduced from Ebnezar J. Textbook of Orthopaedics: with clinical examination methods in orthopaedics. Delhi: Jaypee Brothers Medical Publishers, 2010.

Figures 13.2a and b are reproduced from: Bapat PS. Arriving at a Surgical Diagnosis. Delhi: Jaypee Brothers Medical Publishers, 2013.

# General principles

## 1.1 Fractures and dislocations

A fracture is a break or loss of continuity in a bone. They are either open or closed, and may involve a joint surface (see below). The mechanism of injury (e.g. pathological, stress, periprosthetic) should be sought because it will give a clue as to the nature of the fracture. There is always a significant soft tissue component of fractures that requires consideration as part of the pattern of injury.

### Types

Fractures are described by (**Figure 1.1**):

- Skin being intact (closed) or not (open)
- How many pieces of bone: two (simple) multiple (comminuted)
- Fracture pattern, e.g. oblique, tranverse, spiral, greenstick
- Anatomical location in the bone, i.e. diaphysis, metaphysis
- Joint involvement (articular) or not (nonarticular)
- Displacement. If displaced, the fracture will be any combination of: translation, angulation, rotation, shortening, distraction

### Closed vs open fracture

An open (compound) fracture is one that communicates with an opening (break) in the skin. Any fracture that involves a body cavity which communicates with the skin, e.g. a pelvic fracture involving the rectum or vagina is also an open fracture.

> ### Guiding principle
>
> A fracture can result from forces that are:
> - Sudden and large – acute trauma such as a car accident
> - Repetitive – e.g. stress fracture
> - Trivial – e.g. pathological fracture

Open fractures have more complications and are often caused by high-energy trauma. They can involve skin loss, injury to nerves and blood vessels, and be contaminated by

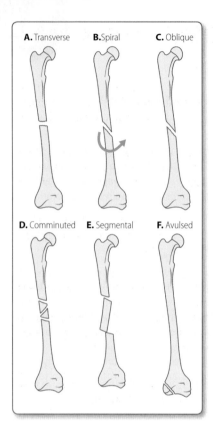

**Figure 1.1** Fracture patterns.

A. Transverse  B. Spiral  C. Oblique

D. Comminuted  E. Segmental  F. Avulsed

debris (e.g. soil). All open fractures require prompt assessment and management to reduce the risks of complications.

## Simple vs comminuted fracture

A simple fracture is a fracture consists of two parts of bone; fractures with more than two parts are comminuted.

## Articular vs nonarticular fracture

Articular fractures involve the surface of a joint; nonarticular fractures do not. Articular fractures require careful management because of the risk of post-traumatic arthrosis, which can occur even after effective treatment.

## Fracture displacement

Displacements are bone deformities caused by a fracture. They are described as the position of the distal fragment relative to the proximal and are usually categorised using radiographs.

**Angulation** Angulation describes the angle that the bone is left at after the fracture. It is given in degrees in either the coronal plane (varus v valgus) and/or the sagittal plane (anterior v posterior).

**Rotation** Rotation describes the angle a bone twists after fracture. It is difficult to determine accurately from a radiograph and is usually more obvious clinically.

**Translation and shortening** Translation is the displacement of the fracture parts away from each other. This distance is estimated and often described using the bone as a reference, e.g. 'translated 50% of the width of the bone'. If the bones are also left overlapping, the length of this overlap is estimated and referred to as shortening.

**Distraction and impaction** Distraction and impaction refer to the distance or overlap, respectively, of two parts of bone after fracture if they are not displaced (i.e. still aligned).

## Dislocations

Dislocations are described by:
- Direction of displacement
- Associated fractures
- Associated injuries, e.g. vascular, neurological

Any joint can be dislocated either by an indirect or direct force. Where there is no congruity between the joint surfaces the joint is dislocated; where there is partial congruity the joint is subluxed.

Neighbouring structures such as ligaments, nerves and blood vessels can all be injured by a dislocation. In some cases the blood vessels are kinked or stretched, compromising the

blood supply distally. This is common in ankle fracture dislocations, but reducing the dislocation restores the blood supply
promptly.

## Healing and complications

Most fractures heal without complications or significant loss
of function. However, complications, which can arise early
or late, have the potential to cause both local and systemic
problems.

The risk of complications is determined by many factors,
both fracture-specific and patient-specific. Fracture-specific
factors include open fractures, comminution, intra-articular
involvement, soft tissue injury and dislocation. Patient-specific
factors include age, weight and comorbidities.

### Bone healing

Bone generally takes 6–8 weeks to heal. The process may take
over a year for full fracture healing and remodelling, but clinically the patient will be asymptomatic. In general terms, most
fractures heal well.

Fracture healing occurs in an environment that encour-
ages the process. The more that environment is respected, the
greater the likelihood of healing.

**Stages of healing**  Fracture healing begins with development
of a haematoma and then proceeds in three stages:
- Inflammation
- Repair
- Remodelling

To optimise healing, there needs to be good anatomical reduction (good bony contact and alignment), immobilisation and
no infection. In other words, the environment for fracture healing has to be correct, taking into account all these factors. The
amount of new bone formed, known as callus, is inversely pro-
portional to the amount of movement across the fracture site.

The haematoma provides haemopoietic cells, which secrete
the necessary growth factors and initiate the inflammatory
stage. Within 2 weeks, primary callus is formed, which is then

converted to hard callus. When the bone ends are not in contact, bridging callus is formed.

In the final stage, the newly formed bone is remodelled to restore the bone's prefracture ability to bear physiological load.

## Local complications

General complications to the site of the fracture occur immediately, early in the healing process (within days) or late (after 6 weeks). Early complications are:
- vascular injury
- soft tissue injury
- compartment syndrome
- infections
- nerve injury

Late complications are:
- delayed union
- non-union
- malunion
- implant complications: infection, prominence, breakage
- joint stiffness
- avascular necrosis
- osteomyelitis
- growth disturbance or arrest
- osteoarthritis
- contractures
- complex regional pain syndrome
- heterotopic ossification

## Systemic complications

General systemic complications affect the body more widely and, like local complications, occur either early or late in the healing process. Early complications are:
- thromboembolism
- pneumonia
- acute respiratory distress syndrome
- acute renal failure
- fat embolism

- shock
- multiorgan failure

Late complications are:
- sepsis
- pressure sores
- muscle wasting
- reduced mobility

## 1.2 Consent

Consent is the permission granted by a patient for a medical procedure, including surgery, to be performed. A surgeon is liable if a patient's consent is not obtained correctly before a procedure is carried out.

Consent must also be obtained for any adjunctive procedures. The patient must be advised of alternate treatment options and the consequences of not undergoing treatment. The complications of, and recovery from, the procedure must be explained and documented. Ideally, consent for the procedure should be taken at the time of admission.

> ### Clinical insight
>
> You should not be expected to ask a patient for their consent to a procedure that you cannot carry out, have not seen carried out or cannot fully explain. In such situations, always ask a senior colleague for advice; in cases of doubt, do not feel obliged to try to obtain a patient's consent.

### Types of consent

There are different types of consent.
- Implied consent is presumed for minor procedures, such as radiography and phlebotomy
- Expressed verbal consent is normally adequate for simple procedures with minimal risk of harm, for example insertion of a nasogastric tube
- Expressed written consent is required for all surgical procedures; written consent is not legal proof that adequate consent has been obtained, but rather proof that a discussion has taken place outlining the specifics of the procedure, risks and benefits, along with the other aspects discussed below

For any consent to be valid, it must be voluntary and informed, and the patient giving it must have capacity.

## Voluntary
The decision to give consent should be the patient's alone; there should be no coercion or pressure from family, friends or medical staff.

## Informed
The patient should be given all the information about the procedure:

- the reason for carrying out the procedure
- what it involves
- the benefits of the procedure
- the risks of the procedure in terms of possible complications
- other treatment options
- the possible consequences if the procedure is not carried out

> ### Clinical insight
> Good communication is key to obtaining consent. Always ask the patient if they have understood what is involved and if there is anything more they would like to know. A translator may be required if the patient does not share your first language.

The patient needs to be fully informed, i.e. no information should be withheld from them.

## Capacity
To give consent, a patient must have capacity, i.e. the ability to make decisions regarding their care. They must be able to:

- understand the information they are given about the procedure
- retain the information
- weigh the risks and benefits of the procedure in order to make a decision whether to agree to it
- communicate their decision

All adults are assumed to have capacity unless there is significant evidence against this. Factors that reduce capacity are:

- dementia
- acute confusion
- mental illness

- intellectual disability
- drug or alcohol intoxication
- use of certain medications
- fatigue

## Capacity assessment

Capacity can change, so it is assessed at the time that consent is required. This is usually at admission for an emergency and at outpatient listing for an elective case. Capacity can be rechecked at any time during the patient's stay. Consent is usually checked verbally at multiple times prior to the patient's procedure.

A patient may have capacity to consent to one procedure but not another. For example, a patient with intellectual disability may be able to give consent for a blood test but may lack the capacity to consent to a procedure with longer term consequences, such as an operation.

> ## Clinical insight
>
> Every hospital has its own specific consent forms. There are usually separate ones for adults with capacity, mentally incapacitated patients and children.

If a patient makes a decision that you consider irrational, their decision will stand as long as they have capacity.

## Lack of capacity

If a patient lacks capacity, decisions about their treatment depend on whether:

- they have made an advance statement or an advance decision to refuse treatment
- they have conferred a lasting power of attorney on another person, giving that person the authority to make decisions on their behalf, should they lose capacity
- an independent mental capacity advocate has been assigned to represent and support the patient

If none of these conditions apply, decisions must be made on behalf of the patient by the doctor responsible for their care.

Any decision made on a patient's behalf must be in their best interests, considering their preferences, wishes, beliefs and values. Whenever possible, the views of the family and friends of the patient should be sought when making such decisions.

### Capacity in children

In most countries, as in the UK, over 16s are regarded as adults and have capacity by default. Under 16s can give consent on their own behalf if they are judged to understand what a treatment involves and its possible consequences (termed Gillick competence).

> ## Clinical insight
>
> In the UK, an advance statement is a written statement of a patient's preferences, wishes, beliefs and values for use as guidance should they lose capacity. It is not legally binding but must be taken into account by those responsible for their care.
>
> An advance decision to refuse treatment, sometimes referred to as an advance directive or living will, is a written statement of a patient's decision to refuse specific treatments should they lose capacity. An advance decision is legally binding.

A child's decision to refuse a treatment, unlike that of an adult, can be overruled by a person with parental responsibility or a court if treatment is deemed to be in the child's best interests.

# Clinical essentials

## 2.1 Common symptoms and how to take a history

Acute or chronic orthopaedic pathology generally causes:
- pain
- swelling
- joint stiffness, often present in degenerative conditions
- loss of function as a result of the combination of pain, deformity and stiffness

The orthopaedic history (**Table 2.1**) focuses on pain, disability and functional loss.

### Common symptoms

#### Pain

Pain is a subjective symptom reported by the patient and the predominant feature in most cases of fracture. The different types of pain gives clues as to the underlying condition, for example:
- painful joints, particularly on movement, are a feature of arthritic conditions
- burning or tingling pains are consistent with neurological disorders
- acute trauma, such as a fracture, sprain or dislocation, will cause severe pain local to the area of trauma

Analgesia is always given to patients experiencing pain postoperatively or in an acute conditions.

#### Swelling

Joint swelling is very common in degenerative skeletal conditions, due to chronic deformity, effusion or generalised thickening of the soft tissues. Differentials include:
- inflammatory arthropathies such as rheumatoid disease
- a large tumour, either in the bone or soft tissues
- acute inflammatory arthritis

| Aspect | Questions |
|---|---|
| Age | – |
| Sex | – |
| Occupation | What is the patient's occupation? Have they stopped work as a consequence of their condition? |
| Presenting complaint | What is the main complaint as experienced by the patient? Pain, swelling, stiffness, numbness, mechanical symptoms? |
| History of presenting complaint | How long has the complaint been present? When did it start? How did it start? How has it progressed? Does the patient use walking aids? Are they able to carry out activities of daily living? |
| Past medical and surgical history | What is the previous history of joint or orthopaedic problems? Any previous orthopaedic interventions? Other medical conditions? |
| Drug history | What analgesics, steroids and disease-modifying antirheumatic drugs does the patient use? |
| Family history | Family history of joint or orthopaedic problems |
| Social history | Where does the patient live? Do they have to use stairs? How has the condition affected their social circumstances? |
| Systems review | Assess overall fitness of patient and confirm underlying conditions impacting on general health |

**Table 2.1** Aspects of the orthopaedic history.

## Joint stiffness

Joint stiffness, like pain, is subjective, so it should be clarified exactly what the patient means. It usually occurs in chronic conditions (e.g. osteoarthrosis) as a consequence of pain through the arc of movement of the joint, manifesting as stiffness or reluctance to move the joint. Joints may also be truly stiff due to a change in their internal architecture as a consequence of gradual deformity, such as that occurring in arthrosis or caused by a malunited intra-articular fracture.

Joint dislocations and fractures around joints cause significant stiffness secondary to the extensive soft tissue injury.

Some conditions that complicate injuries, such as heterotopic ossification, also cause joints to stiffen.

### Joint stiffness after injury

Joint stiffness can occur in the short-, medium- or long-term period after injury (**Table 2.2**). It is also the common end point of many chronic arthritic conditions.

> ## Guiding principle
>
> Fractures involving joints, i.e. intra-articular fractures, are at greater risk of leading to post-traumatic stiffness and arthritis. Joint immobilisation allows the fracture to heal, but early joint movement is also necessary to to prevent stiffness. A secure and stable internal fixation of allows an early controlled range of motion that mitigates against joint stiffness.

Most joints have a range of movement that exceeds day-to-day requirements, so some loss as a result of stiffness is tolerated. However, problems arise when the reduction in range of movement impairs function, for example when restricted elbow flexion makes it difficult for patients to feed themselves. Early intervention can prevent long-term joint stiffness.

## Loss of function

The degree of loss of function as a result of an injury depends on the nature of the injury, subsequent stiffness and muscle atrophy. Muscle atrophy occurs when muscles are not actively contracting; eventually they lose volume which may never fully recover. This process is initiated by pain and/or immobilisation. For example, quadriceps mass starts to diminish 48 hours after a knee injury. Functional outcome is usually improved by

| Time frame | Cause | Prevention |
|---|---|---|
| Short term | Pain, swelling, apprehension | Anatomical reduction, appropriate splintage |
| Medium term | Temporary stiffness after immobilisation | Early movement, early referral to physiotherapy |
| Long term | Permanent muscle and tendon shortening, arthritis | Physiotherapy, adaptations, orthoses, surgical releases |

**Table 2.2** Joint stiffness: causes and prevention

physiotherapy and exercise but not necessarily restored to the preinjury level of function.

Loss of function can be caused by transient or permanent neurological injury. About 40% of bone and joint injuries include peripheral nerve lesions leading to a sensory deficit, motor function deficit or both (**Table 2.3**).

## Structure of the orthopaedic history

In the context of acute trauma, the history is used to elicit the mechanism of injury, energy involved and time elapsed between injury and presentation. Non-traumatic orthopaedic disease includes arthritic conditions, congenital conditions, nerve entrapments, soft tissue conditions and functional problems. They are assessed using a logical sequence of inquiry to obtain the presenting complaint and explore its history.

### Age

Certain injuries and diseases are associated with specific age groups (**Tables 2.4** and **2.5**).

| Type of nerve injury | Seddon class | Cause | Prognosis |
|---|---|---|---|
| Neuropraxia | I | Compression | Good full recovery |
| Axonotmesis | II | Injury to the axon, with intact epineurium | Guarded recovery occurs over many years |
| | III | Type II with endoneurium injury | |
| | IV | Type II with perineurium injury | |
| Neurotmesis | V | Complete disruption of nerve trunk | Poor; full recovery unlikely, surgical intervention is needed |

**Table 2.3** Seddon classification of peripheral nerve injury.

| Stage of life | Cause of trauma | Example injuries |
|---|---|---|
| Birth | Birth, traumatic delivery | Brachial plexus injury, clavicular fracture, humeral fracture |
| Early childhood (0–3 years) | Fall while learing to walk | Metaphyseal/diaphyseal fracture of the tibia (toddler fracture) |
| | Non accidental injury | Multiple rib fractures, metaphyseal fractures |
| Late childhood (3–12 years) | Fall, e.g. from trampoline | Posterior dislocation of elbow |
| | Repeated loading in the obese child | Slipped capital femoral epiphysis |
| | Fall from a height | Monteggia fracture, supracondylar fracture of humerus |
| Adolescence | Fall on outstretched hand (from height) | Upper limb and clavicular fractures |
| Adulthood | Fall from height | Upper limb and spine injuries, pilon fracture, calcaneal fracture |
| | Diving | Cervical spine injury |
| | Road traffic accident | Any combination |
| | | Whiplash injury (injury to tendons and ligaments of neck from sudden forward, backward or sideways movement of head) |
| | | Dashboard injuries (e.g. patellar fracture, posterior hip dislocation) |
| | Sports | Ankle, shoulder, knee and elbow injuries |
| | Assault | Long bone fracture |
| Old age | Trivial fall | Distal radius, humeral neck fracture |
| | | Neck-of-femur fracture |

**Table 2.4** Trauma and injury at different stages of life.

| Age (years) | Disease |
|---|---|
| < 1 | Developmental dysplasia of the hip (DDH) and cerebral palsy |
| 1–2 | Nutritional rickets |
| | Poliomyelitis |
| 3–10 | Tuberculosis of hip, septic arthritis, discitis |
| | Perthes' disease, transient synovitis |
| 10–20 | Slipped capital epiphysis, tarsal coalition, Osgood–Schlatter's disease, recurrent patellar dislocation |
| < 15 | Osteomyelitis |
| 30–40 | Rheumatoid arthritis |
| > 40 | Degenerative disorders |
| | Prolapsed intervertebral disc |
| | Multiple myeloma, secondary/metastatic bone tumour |

**Table 2.5** Orthopaedic diseases commonly presenting in different age groups.

## Sex

Perthes' disease, slipped capital femoral epiphysis, traumatic disorders and multiple myeloma are more common in men. Girls and women present with more cases of developmental dysplasia of the hip, rheumatoid arthritis and osteoporosis.

## Occupation

A patient's occupation is relevant to the cause of their condition, ability to return to work and treatment choice. For example:

- patients with arthritic conditions struggle with manual labour or jobs requiring prolonged standing
- athletes with chronic ankle or knee injuries are likely to have osteoarthrosis in the long term
- arthoplasty surgery can be career-ending for patient whose jobs involve manual labour

Consideration is given to the type of surgery and approach, to avoid impacting too much on patient's work. For example, an anterior approach to the knee for a tibial nail is always associated with inability to kneel, a consideration that will be important to a carpet fitter with a tibial shaft fracture.

## Presenting complaint

The most common presenting complaints are:

- pain
- stiffness
- swelling
- instability
- functional loss

**Pain**  The patient is asked to estimate the severity of their pain on a scale of 1–10, with 10 being the most severe pain they have ever experienced (**Figure 2.1**). Periodic reassessments of pain are used to measure improvement and the effectiveness of any intervention.

The SOCRATES mnemonic summarises the features to note when eliciting a full history of pain.

- Site
- Onset
- Character
- Radiation
- Associations
- Timings

> ## Clinical insight
>
> Fracture pain is exacerbated by movement and muscle spasm. Early immobilisation with a splint, a non-circumferential rigid material that allows swelling, helps control pain.

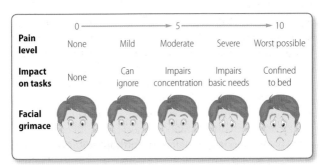

**Figure 2.1** Scale of severity of pain.

- Exacerbating features
- Severity

**Stiffness**   Stiffness is the feeling of having trouble moving a joint. Ask how long the patient has been stiff and if there was an injury. Assess if there is difference between active (patient moves themselves) and passive (joint is moved for the patient) range of movement.

**Swelling**   Swelling is an enlargement of an area due to fluid accumulation. Ask how long it has been present, if it is exacerbated by exercise and if it has got worse.

**Instability**   Ask if the joint gives way without warning and if the patient trusts the joint. Establish if pain is the predominant feature giving rise to instability and if there are any mechanical symptoms, such as locking.

## History of presenting complaint

The history of the presenting complaint describes the mechanism of injury, including the energy and direction of force, as well as the time of injury. The energy of the injury must be considered and determined; it is either direct or indirect. The level of energy and mode of trauma suggest certain fracture patterns and associated injuries. For example, high-energy injuries are associated with greater incidence and severity of complications and degree of soft tissue damage than low-energy injuries.

> ### Guiding principle
>
> Trauma is the event that causes the injury. The injury is the combination of pathological changes in tissue structure and function caused by the trauma.

**Events surrounding trauma**   A careful history is taken of events surrounding the trauma, particularly symptoms indicating an underlying medical condition. For example, chest pain suggests angina or myocardial infarction, and numbness or weakness suggests a cerebrovascular accident.

Significant medical conditions must be identified and their management optimised before any orthopaedic intervention. Specialist advice is sought, if necessary.

The underlying medical condition may require the patient to be admitted to hospital under shared care, or even to a high-dependency or critical care ward. Surgery, if otherwise indicated, may be postponed or cancelled indefinitely if the risks of operating outweigh any benefits.

**Falls** Orthopaedic injuries, especially in the elderly, are frequently caused by falls. The cause, for example an acute medical problem such as a vasovagal collapse, cerebrovascular accident or cardiac event, must be determined whenever possible. A range of transient conditions, such as urinary tract infections or dehydration, give rise to dizziness or unconsciousness, causing the patient to fall. Frail patients with poor balance are prone to repeated falls.

## Past medical and surgical history

A review of the patient's medical and surgical history is essential to ascertain any previous injuries or surgery that will impact on surgical decision making. It is useful to know whether there are any conditions or medications that may have increased the likelihood or severity of injury, for example osteoporosis or the use of steroids. Poor wound healing and susceptibility to infection are often secondary to certain medical conditions, such as diabetes, peripheral neuropathies and vascular disease.

## Drug history

All drugs have some bearing on patients' fitness for surgery. Remember to always prescribe the patient's regular medication, such as antihypertensives, when they are admitted.

Ask about the patient's history of analgesic medication (including its frequency), whether it is adequate and whether the patient take it regularly or as required. Cytotoxics, steroids and disease-modifying agents for rheumatoid disease (DMARDS) all affect healing and should be asked about. Ask about illicit drug use, including steroids because these can cause comorbidities. Also consider drugs that are directly associated with a condition, such as quinolone antibiotics (associated with achilles tendon rupture).

## Family history

Ask about any condition that might be relevant to the presenting complaint. For example, Charcot–Marie–Tooth disease is a hereditary sensory motor neuropathy that causes muscular dystrophy and patients with osteogenesis imperfecta have brittle bones.

Conditions such as type 2 diabetes and cardiovascular disease also have a genetic components, and impact on patients' fitness for surgery.

## Social history

Information about where the patient lives and who is at home to support them affects the treatment options available, timing and nature of surgery, and the patient's ability to return to work and their previous activities. Specifically, ask about:
- stairs: either within, or to gain access to, the house
- easily accessible bathrooms
- whether the patient drives
- any hobbies

## Systems review

A systems review includes assessment of:
- general symptoms: weight loss, fatigue, lethargy, night sweats, appetite, fever
- cardiovascular symptoms: chest pain, shortness of breath, palpitations, orthopnoea, claudication
- respiratory symptoms: cough, sputum, wheeze, haemoptysis, shortness of breath
- gastrointestinal symptoms: abdominal pain, difficulty in swallowing, weight loss, nausea, vomiting, diarrhoea, constipation
- neurological symptoms: special senses, fits, seizures, balance problems

All of these assess the general fitness of the patient, along with other conditions that may need investigating prior to any orthopaedic intervention.

| Disease | Features |
|---------|----------|
| Congenital | Present since birth or seen within a few years from birth; strong family history |
| Developmental | Manifests during childhood or adolescence |
| Infective | Fever, chills, rigors, sweating |
| Inflammatory | Seasonal variation, remissions and exacerbation, multiple joint involvement |
| Metabolic | Nutritional factors, low socioeconomic status, generalised skeletal disorder |
| Hormonal | Hormonal imbalance (e.g. congenital hypothyroidism leading to cretinism, and hypopituitarism to dwarfism) |
| Trauma | History of a fall, road traffic accident, assault, etc. |
| Degenerative | Advancing age, slow progression |
| Neoplastic | Features of benign or malignant bone tumours (e.g. pathological fractures; cachexia; history or features of breast, prostate, lung, kidney or thyroid cancer) |

**Table 2.6** Pathological categories of orthopaedic disease and their features.

## Diagnostic categories

Other than in obvious cases of trauma, the information from the history should inform a tentative diagnosis (**Table 2.6**) and help focus the examination.

# 2.2 Clinical signs and examination

The goal of orthopaedic examination, informed by thorough history-taking, is to assess and describe any musculoskeletal abnormalities present. This provides a provisional diagnosis to guide the choice of investigations. Function is assessed by observing the patient while they are examined (e.g. when walking or getting dressed) and specific abnormalities are defined by special tests. Gait, i.e. a person's pattern of walking, also informs diagnosis in cases of spinal, hip and lower limb disorders.

## Clinical signs

The key signs seen in orthopaedic examination are alignment, deformity, swelling, tenderness, restricted movement and abnormalities of gait and function.

## Tenderness

Tenderness is pain elicited by palpation. Specific, targeted palpation elicits the structures involved in any pathology. Tenderness is often a very sensitive indicator of the precise location of the problem. It may be the only evidence of fracture in cases of:

- crack fracture
- stress fracture
- torus fracture
- pathological fracture

## Deformities

Deformities are deviations of the normal anatomy of a bone or joint, or both (**Table 2.7**). Always compare the injured side with the contralateral side, but bear in mind this may not be normal either.

| Region | Sign | Definition |
|--------|------|------------|
| Spine and neck | Torticollis | Twisting of the neck to one side |
| | Scoliosis | Lateral spinal curvature in the coronal plane |
| Upper limb | Winging of the scapula | Abnormal protrusion of the scapula |
| Hand and wrist | Bouchard's nodes | Osteoarthritic enlargement of the PIP joints |
| | Heberden's nodes | Osteoarthritic enlargement of the DIP joints |
| | Mallet finger | Isolated flexion at the DIP joint |
| | Claw hand | Extension at the MCP joints with flexion at the DIP and PIP joints |

**Table 2.7** Common orthopaedic deformities. *Continues overleaf*

| Region | Sign | Definition |
|--------|------|------------|
| | Swan neck deformity | Extension at the PIP joint and flexion at the PIP joint |
| | Boutonnière deformity | Flexion of the PIP joints with hyperflexion of the DIP joints |
| | Ulnar deviation of the fingers | Medial deviation of the fingers at the level of the MCP joints |
| | Caput ulna | Prominence of the ulna at the wrist as a result of subluxation and palmar translation of the radius at the distal radioulnar joint |
| Hip | Fixed flexion deformity | Inability of the affected hip to reach full extension |
| Knee | Genu valgum | A knocked knee deformity; lateral deviation of the tibia |
| | Genu varum | A bow-legged deformity; medial deviation of the tibia |
| Foot and ankle | Hindfoot varus | Angling of the heel towards the midline as viewed from behind |
| | Hindfoot valgus | Excessive angling of the heel away from the midline as viewed from behind |
| | Pes planus | Loss of the medial arch |
| | Pes cavus | Exaggeration of the medial arch |
| | Hallux valgus (bunion) | Lateral deviation of the great toe |
| | Hallux rigidus | Stiffness of the great toe MTP joint |
| | Claw toes | Hyperextension at the MTP joint with flexion at the PIP and DIP joints |
| | Hammertoes | Flexion at the PIP joint |
| | Mallet toe | Flexion at the DIP joint |

DIP, distal interphalangeal; MCP, metacarpophalangeal; MTP, metatarsophalangeal; PIP, proximal interphalangeal.

**Table 2.7** *Continued*

## Joint posture

Joint posture is described in the coronal, sagittal and axial planes. In the coronal plane:

- valgus: the distal part of the limb angles away from the midline, e.g. genu valgum (knock-knee)
- varus: the distal part of the limb angles towards the midline, e.g. genu varum (bow-leg)

In the sagittal plane a joint is either flexed or extended, while the axial plan describes the deformity. All deformities are either fixed, correctable or partially correctable. Any limb or digit can also be short or long, compared to the normal side.

## Scars

Scars indicate a previous injury: either traumatic or planned surgical incision. The site, extent (regular or irregular) and age should be described. Scars can give information on a previous injury or the type of operation performed. For example, a longitudinal mid-line incision over the front of the knee indicates a previous knee arthroplasty. Afro-Caribbean and South Asian populations are particularly prone to keloid scarring.

## Asymmetry

Asymmetry should be checked for in other parts of the examination, including gait, limb alignment, scars, muscle bulk and skin creases.

## Muscle wasting or weakness

This represents atrophy of myocytes as a consequence of lack of use. Causes of this include:

- CNS causes, e.g. Guillain–Barré
- injury to, or neurological conditions of, peripheral nerves
- direct injury to the muscle
- multisystemic conditions, e.g. cachexia

Look for the extent and location of wasting; is it generalised or localised? Test for any consequent weakness and describe the muscle contours.

## Colour

Vitiligo is the loss of skin pigmentation. Redness (erythema) over limbs and joints indicates infection. Jaundice (yellowing) indicates liver disease.

## Type of swelling

Swelling can be local or diffuse. Establish if there is generalised soft tissue swelling or an effusion, and if there is any associated pain or tenderness. Generalised swelling indicates a systemic disease, such as congestive cardiac failure. Unilateral calf swelling is often the only evidence of a deep vein thrombosis.

**Joint effusion** Effusion can occur in any joint secondary to trauma, inflammation or infection. It is more obvious in superficial joints, e.g. the knee, ankle, wrist and fingers, than in deep joints, e.g. the shoulder and hip. An ultrasound or trial aspiration will confirm the presence of an effusion in joints other than the knee. Knee effusions are often palpable.

## Bruising

Bruising is caused either by direct trauma or small tears under the skin for a more distant injury. Bruises are red initially, then fade to a yellow/brown after 2 weeks. Patients on anticoagulants and the elderly are more prone to bruising. Blood collecting under the skin and causing swelling is a haematoma. Always ensure the overlying skin is still intact.

## Rashes

Rashes are not common orthopaedic problems, but are seen as side effects of antibiotics and other medicines, and effects of other diseases, including some that involve the musculoskeletal system. For example, psoriatic plaques indicate active disease that help diagnose psoriatic arthropathy. Conditions such as psoriasis and eczema are optimised prior to surgery because incisions through skin lesions have a higher risk of infection. Rashes may also indicate a more systemic pathology that might require investigation at first presentation.

## Wounds

Wounds, like scars, are either the result of surgery or trauma. Assess traumatic wounds for depth, regularity, extent, site and degree of contamination. The wound may also be part of an open fracture picture. Often, such wounds undergo delayed primary or secondary closure.

Surgical wounds present as a problem after the patient has been discharged following surgery. In general, wounds over an arthroplasty are discussed with the operating surgeon because any injudicious use of antibiotics can compromise future treatment should a deep infection ensue. It is important to identify and treat a superficial infection.

> ### Clinical insight
>
> Limb ischaemia suggested by the five P's:
> * pain
> * pallor
> * paraesthesia
> * pulselessness
> * paralysis

### Other signs of injury or chronic change

Many diseases relevant to orthopaedics have cutaneous manifestations, e.g. café-au-lait spots in neurofibromatosis, haemosiderin deposits in chronic venous insufficiency and lipodermatosclerosis in diabetes. Look for any ulceration: either vascular, neuropathic and/or mixed. Look for sinuses, check for pulses distal to the pathology and assess neurological function.

**Joint crepitus** This is an abnormal grating sensation either felt or heard in cases of displaced fracture or degenerative joint conditions. It is caused by friction between two irregular surfaces.

> ### Clinical insight
>
> Do not specifically attempt to elicit crepitus in an acute fracture. This does not aid the diagnosis and will cause undue pain to the patient.

**Fixed flexion** Fixed flexion is a joint that does not return to the extended position. If it can be passively corrected this is an extensor lag. Most fixed flexion deformities (FFD) are caused by trauma to the joint, such as a fracture or soft tissue trauma. Arthritis over time and contracture of muscle also cause flexion deformities.

The cause can be difficult to determine. Painful acute fixed flexion of the knee (locking) is almost always caused by a meniscal tear. FFDs are described in degrees: if the FFD is 15° then a deficit of 15° is needed to return the joint to the extended position.

**Restricted range of movement** Restricted range of motion implies both restriction in extension and flexion (like fixed flexion), and is either permanent or temporary. For example, acute trauma causes a temporary restriction in joint range due to pain.

Test the range of motion actively and passively; comment on the arc of movement (in degrees) and if that arc provides any function.

Soft tissue contractures, heterotopic ossification, and intra-articular trauma all cause permanent restricted range of movement. An acute, hot, red joint with severely restricted range of active and passive range of motion suggests septic arthritis and requires urgent investigation.

**Joint swelling** Joint swelling is always pathological. Note the distribution of the swelling: does it involve one joint or many? Is it symmetrical? Symmetrical joint swelling is often due to an inflammatory condition that affects multiple joints, such as rheumatoid arthritis or osteoarthritis. Conditions such as gout tend to affect one joint only.

**Warmth** Heat or warmth in any joint suggests an inflammatory process caused by either an acute or chronic condition, e.g. gout or osteoarthritis. Septic arthritis presents as a hot swollen joint that can mimic other arthritic conditions. Urgent aspiration and a gram stain are required to exclude this diagnosis.

## Orthopaedic examination
The generic orthopaedic examination comprises:
- inspection (i.e. look)
- palpation (i.e. feel)
- elicitation of both active and passive movement (i.e. move)
- measurement of the length and girth of the limb
- special tests

### Traumatic versus non-traumatic examination

In trauma patients the priority is to identify and treat life- and limb-threatening injuries in a timely fashion. Orthopaedic injuries are identified and defined quickly, along with any neurovascular compromises. The patient is examined from head to toe to look for an injury. The patient cannot assist with this if they are unconscious, and a neurological examination will not be possible. Pain often distracts from less significant injuries. In cases of acute trauma, life-threatening injuries or conditions are managed before examination of non-life threatening orthopaedic injuries.

Outside of the acute setting patients often present with a single problem and there is time to take a thorough history and specific examination.

### General examination

Vital sign assessment and cardiovascular, respiratory, abdominal and neurological screening examinations are carried out as a quick assessment. A general screening examination is particularly important if surgery is being considered, and is usually done after the orthopaedic examination. Junior doctors often perform this examination to identify treatable abnormalities.

### Beginning the examination

After consent has been obtained, the patient is asked to remove their clothing to expose the area in question as well as the joint above and below it. The contralateral side must also be exposed to allow assessment of symmetry.

### Gait

The patient is observed walking with or without aids, as required, from behind, in front and the side. They are observed turning. Features of their gait may suggest a diagnosis (**Table 2.8**). The patient is also observed for spinal deformities (**Figure 2.2**).

### Joint examination

Examination of each joint follows the order of 'Look, feel and move'.

| Gait | Feature | Cause |
|------|---------|-------|
| Antalgic gait | Stance phase decreased | Any painful lesion of the hip, knee, ankle or foot |
| High-stepping gait | High step required to keep dropped foot clear of ground | Foot drop |
| Scissor gait | Legs cross while walking | Cerebral palsy |
| Short leg gait | Pelvis dips down on affected side | Limb shortening (congenital or acquired) |
| Stiff hip gait | No flexion at hip | Hip pathology, including infection, tuberculosis |
| Quadriceps gait | Limping gait with hand on knee | Poliomyelitis |
| Trendelenburg gait | Pelvis drops on opposite side to affected hip | Weakness of the abductor muscles caused by chronic osteoarthritis |
| Calcaneal gait | No push-off | Calf weakness |
| Stiff knee gait | Pelvis raised during swing phase | Stiff knee |
| Ataxic gait | Wide-based gait, unsteady | Cerebellar disease |

**Table 2.8** Types of gait and their cause.

**Look**  Look at the affected joint and the contralateral side. Assess for the following.
- Deformities (see **Table 2.7**): describe the joint deformity and its correctability
- Posture of the joint: is it in a flexed or extended position? Is it correctable?
- Scars: describe their nature, site and age. Is there multiple scarring? Measure the length of the scar and assess its tenderness
- Asymmetry: look for overall asymmetry in posture and gait with the patient standing. Look for asymmetry of movement at joints, actively and passively

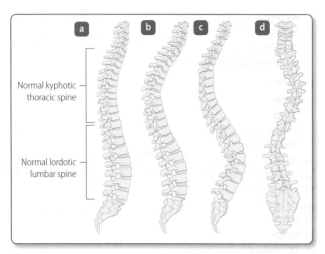

**Figure 2.2** Spinal anomolies. (a) Normal, (b) kyphosis, (c) lordosis and (d) scoliosis.

- Muscle wasting: inspect from the front, the side and behind the patient. Measure muscle bulk circumferentially with a tape measure on both sides from a fixed bony point
- Colour: observe colour changes to the limbs. Is it local or diffuse?
- Swelling: is localised or diffuse? Specifically related to a joint or multiple joints? Palpate the swelling to define its nature: effusion, lipoma, bony swelling, cystic
- Bruising: document size, site and colour. Look and palpate for haematoma. Comment on the quality of the overlying skin; is there necrosis?
- Rashes: define extent and shape. Note any infection or breaks. If chronic, the patient may offer an opinion on diagnosis
- Wounds: observe site and age. Are they surgical or traumatic? Any evidence of infection? Any sutures that need removing? Any other concerns such as gaping or dehisscence?
- Other signs of injury or chronic change: Look for other markers of chronic disease. Note ulcers or skin changes consistent

with chronic venous insufficiency. Do they require walking aids or splints? Is the gait normal? Is there pain when walking? Are there orthotics in their shoes? Is one limb shorter? Is the gait steady or unbalanced?

**Feel**  First, palpate the surface for:

- evenness
- temperature of the joint
- sensation, either reduced (hypoesthesia) or increased (hyperesthesia)

Superficial palpation is followed by deep palpation; the soft tissues, bones and joint space are assessed for how they are arranged and the presence of tenderness. For better patient compliance, palpation proceeds from the normal area to the affected part.

> ### Guiding principle
>
> Know the regional skeletal and soft tissue anatomy of the region you are examining so that you can visualise differences in your mind. Practise, practise, practise on peers.

During palpation, the normal anatomical arrangements are considered and the patient's face is observed to ensure that the assessment is not causing pain.

Swelling and lesions have certain characteristics that help make a clinical diagnosis:

- Is it bony? Note size and site. Is it smooth or irregular, near a joint, tender? The most common bony lesion is an exostosis (benign, bony outgrowth near joint). Others represent calluses from a healing fractures or benign bony conditions to bone malignancy
- Is it superficial or deep? Subcutaneous lesions are generally superficial. If they are deep or tethered to muscle they can be felt by asking the patient to contract underlying muscle
- Is it within the soft tissues? Many lesions, such as nerve sheath tumours and abcesses, are localised to the soft tissues
- Is it within the joint space? Define intra-articular pathology. Torn meniscus and joint space in arthritis are tender to palpation. A meniscal ganglion arises from the intra-articular space
- Is it diffuse or discrete? Is the lesion is well circumscribed. Does it have an outline? Diffusely- or irregularly-shaped?

- Is it tender to palpation? Note any tenderness, tender swelling or discrete lesions
- Is it warm?
- Is it fluctuant. Grasp lesion is gently between thumb and index finger, press on lesion with a third digit. This causes a bulging which is palpable by the examining hand. Lesion contains fluid if this occurs in two perpendicular angles
- Any overlying skin changes? Look for ulcers, sinus, wounds, scars and colour. Induration implies a pointing abcess
- Does the area transilluminate, i.e. the whole lesion will glow when a bright narrow light is shone on it in a darkened room

**Move**  The range of movement of the joint is assessed.

- Ask the patient to move the joint to assess their active range of movement; movements may have to be demonstrated or described explicitly
- Assess the passive range of movement of each joint by moving the joint through its full range with the patient relaxed
- Observe for symmetry and restriction in the range of movement
- Assess for fixed flexion
- Note any pain elicited in the range of movement; observe the patient's face for discomfort. If in doubt, ask the patient if you are hurting them while the joints are being moved
- Test for stability in the coronal and sagittal planes by performing tests that stress each ligament under tension

Special tests are carried out to assess for specific joint abnormalities (**Table 2.9**).

**Clinical insight**

Passive movement is done by the patient; active movement is that done by another person. The passive range of movement is more than the active range in certain axes.

**Guiding principle**

Restricted movements are described as the joint 'lacking the last X degrees of X movement'. For example, an elbow with 20–165° of movement 'lacks the last 20° of extension'.

**Anatomical measurements**

Limbs are measured to assess for shortening. This is

| Joint | Special test | Description |
|-------|-------------|-------------|
| Shoulder | Scarf test for ACJ pathology | With elbow at 90°, take hand to contralateral shoulder. Pain indicates ACJ pathology |
| Wrist | Phalen's test for carpal tunnel syndrome | Fully flex the wrist for 30 s. If pain and paraesthesia occur, test is positive |
| Hip | Thomas's test for fixed flexion deformity at hip | Examine patient supine on couch. Contralateral hip is flexed with examiner's hand placed under lumbar spine. Hip flexion eliminates lumbar lordosis (confirmed) with hand under spine. Hips observed from the side. Any fixed flexion of hip will be seen |
| | True and apparent leg lengths | Examine patient supine on couch with both limbs in similar posture. Measure for true length from anterior superior iliac spine to medial malleolus. Measure for apparent length from umbilicus or xiphisternum to medial malleolus |
| | Trendelenburg's test for hip abduction | Stand in front of standing patient they place their hands on your outstretched hands. They lift their good leg off floor (i.e. stand on affected leg). Abductor weakness causes pelvis to dip or sag away from affected hip. Examiner feels pressure on hand opposite affected hip |
| Knee | Anterior drawer test for ACL damage | Patient is supine with hips flexed to 45°, knees to 90° and feet flat. Sit on patient's toes to stabilise legs. Grasp just below tibiofemoral joint line and try to translate lower leg anteriorly. Positive test if lack of end feel or excessive anterior translation relative to contralateral side |
| | Lachman's test for ACL damage | Flex patient's knee to 30° while they lie supine. One hand behind tibia and the other fixing patient's thigh. Pull tibia forwards. Intact ACL prevents forward moment. If ACL ruptured, tibia translates forwards, often without firm 'end point' |

**Table 2.9** Bedside tests of joint function. *Continues opposite*

| Joint | Special test | Description |
|-------|-------------|-------------|
| Ankle | Calf squeeze test (Simmonds' test or Thompson's test) for Achilles tendon rupture | Patient lies prone with foot off the end of the bed. Squeeze calf. Foot plantar flexes if Achilles tendon intact. No movement indicates rupture |
|       | Anterior drawer test, for ATFL pathology | Patient seated with knee flexed and leg hanging over the couch. Examiner's hand fixes tibia. The other hand is placed behind heel and pulls foot forwards on tibia. Excessive translation of foot compared with normal side indicates laxity of ATFL |

ACJ, acromioclavicular joint; ACL, anterior cruciate ligament; ATFL, anterior talofibular ligament.

**Table 2.9** *Continued*

performed with the patient supine on a couch. Measure before palpating and checking movement, but after you have watched the patient walk and inspected them. Limbs are measured with a tape measure using the same points on either side to allow comparison.

**True and apparent leg lengths**  With the patient supine and their limbs straight, the distance from the greater trochanter and the umbilicus to the medial malleolus is measured (**Figure 2.3**).
- The distance between the trochanter and the medial malleolus is the true leg length
- The distance between the umbilicus and the medial malleolus is the apparent leg length

**Calf and thigh circumference**  A tape measure is used to measure the calf and thigh at the same distance on each leg for comparison above and below the knee. This provides useful information on possible swelling (increased circumference) or muscle wasting (reduced circumference).

**Arm span**  The shoulders are abducted to 90° and the distance between the tips of the middle fingers is measured. In adults,

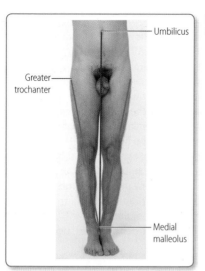

Umbilicus

Greater trochanter

Medial malleolus

**Figure 2.3** True (blue) and apparent (red) leg lengths.

the normal arm span is about 5 cm greater than the person's height. An arm span greater than this can indicate Marfan's syndrome or age-related height loss.

## Fracture and dislocation assessment
A fracture or dislocation (see pages 1–6) is diagnosed based on the presence of pain, tenderness to palpation, swelling and deformity, as well as confirmation on radiography. Movement may be limited, especially if the bone is discontinuous, although some movement usually remains.

## Acute trauma assessment and management
Trauma management is carried out, in accordance with the Advanced Trauma Life Support protocol, to identify and manage life-threatening conditions before examination for less urgent musculoskeletal injuries. Life-threatening orthopaedic injuries include haemorrhage from an open femoral fracture. The limbs are examined as part of the secondary survey.

## Neurovascular status

Traumatic orthopaedic examination includes examination of the neurovascular status of the limb, particularly distal to the zone of injury, and the contralateral side. This documents any progression and/or improvement, and it is mandatory to record this prior to any intervention that will alter nerve function.

- Test the sensory function of the peripheral nerves to the limb, comparing with the contralateral side: note the nerves and distributions tested and the findings
- Test initially using gross touch: establish what is normal by testing an area away from the injury (often the face). Then confirm normal sensation on the uninjured limb. Test all the peripheral nerve sensory distributions distal to the injury, comparing the normal to the injured side
- Test for peripheral nerves, not dermatomes, because limb trauma injures specific nerves
- Test for individual muscle function over the affected joint (or joints) innervated by the same peripheral nerves; this finding is less reliable in the presence of pain, because the patient may be reluctant to move the extremity
- Look at the colour of the skin: pallor indicates vascular compromise
- Test for capillary return; > 2 s suggests sluggish return as a result of the patient being either peripherally shut down as a consequence of shock or an injury to a proximal vessel. Vessels kink or stretch around joint dislocations
- Palpate the named arteries proximal and distal to the injury
- Palpate the same arteries on the contralateral side

---

### Clinical insight

A deformity in the presence of a pale pulseless extremity, for example a dislocated ankle fracture, indicates immediate reduction of the injury with analgesia to restore perfusion distal to the fracture.

- Carry out reduction immediately; do not wait for imaging
- Once alignment and pulses have improved, splint the reduced joint
- Obtain the radiograph
- Finally, recheck neurovascular status

## 2.3 Investigations

Investigations are carried out to identify, define and monitor the progress of an injury or a condition.

### Imaging

Imaging provides evidence leading to a diagnosis. It is not the guiding principle for treatment.

The commonest investigation is plain radiography, an excellent way of imaging fractures, dislocations and bony alignment. Small, superficial joints are visualised more closely with US for certain indications, and MRI is very good for detecting pathological joint changes.

Computerised tomography provides more information on bony injury. It improves anatomical assessment of injuries, particularly intra-articular fractures. A CT scan is helpful when planning fixation of complex fractures. US and MRI scans are more helpful in the assessment of soft tissue injury rather than acute bony injury.

> **Clinical insight**
>
> Any imaging request must contain patient identifiers: the side and site to be imaged must be specified, along with the presumed diagnosis. For plain radiology, specify the films required, e.g. anteroposterior or lateral. If in doubt, ask a radiographer or radiologist.

### Radiography

Radiographs are excellent aids for the diagnosis of most fractures, subluxations and dislocations. They are generally sufficient for the diagnosis of osteoarthritis and for planning the management of most fractures.

At least two views of the area in question are always requested, including views of the joints above and below the injury. The minimum is an anteroposterior and a lateral radiograph.

Postoperative radiographs confirm the nature of the intervention and may be used to monitor progress.

**Principles** Radiographs are produced when X-rays pass through a part of the body and are captured on a film or imaging plate. The image on the film is a shadow of the substances that block X-rays to different degrees depending on their den-

## Clinical insight

Remember the rule of twos for radiographs:

- two planes, to show the bone in two planes
- two joints, both ends of the bones
- two sides; in some cases, radiographs of both limbs or both sides are obtained and compared to help identify the underlying pathology

## Clinical insight

Over-reliance on investigations is no substitute for adequate clinical assessment. When requesting an investigation, consider what information will be obtained and how that will influence treatment.

sity. Denser substances, such as bone, block the passage of X-rays, resulting in a paler area on the film. Conversely, softer tissues allow more X-rays to pass through them, resulting in a dark area on the film.

**Terminology** Substances are described as radiolucent or radiopaque.

- X-rays pass through radiolucent substances with little attenuation and are therefore almost entirely invisible on X-ray
- radiopaque substances are relatively resistant to the passage of X-rays

**Advantages** Radiography can produce an image of most body parts. It is easily available, even by the bedside, in the emergency department and in operating theatres.

**Disadvantages** Radiography provides limited information on soft tissue. Patients and technicians are exposed to low doses of radiation, but the risk is usually outweighed by the utility of the technique in fracture management (**Table 2.11**).

### Computerised tomography

Computerised tomography provides good visualisation of bone and discrimination between different tissue types, even those with similar densities. It produces detailed three-dimensional images of a structure.

**Principles** Multiple thin beams of X-rays are passed through the body from multiple angles (usually > 180°). An array of detectors on the opposite side from the beam measure the amount of X-ray attenuation.

**Terminology** Substances are described as isodense, hypodense or hyperdense.

- Isodense substances have a density similar to that of an adjacent or other tissue (e.g. in the case of isodense subdural haematoma)
- Hypodense substances appear less dense than the surrounding tissue (e.g. fat is hypodense when compared with bone on a CT image)
- Hyperdense substances appear denser than adjacent tissue (e.g. fresh blood is hyperdense)

**Advantages** Computerised tomography is relatively inexpensive compared with MRI. It produces accurate, three-dimensional data including information on attenuation, and data acquisition is rapid.

**Disadvantages** This technique exposes patients to a relatively high amount of ionising radiation per scan (see **Table 2.10**), and is subject to artefacts caused by patient movement. IV contrast is required for certain structures (e.g. vessels), which carries a risk of anaphylaxis.

| Study | Equivalent period of natural background radiation | Estimated additional lifetime risk of cancer per study |
|---|---|---|
| Radiography of extremity | A few hours to a few days | Negligible: < 1 in 1,000,000 |
| Radiography of hip, spine, abdomen or pelvis CT of head | A few months to a year | 1 in 100,000 to 1 in 10,000 |
| CT of chest or abdomen | A few years | 1 in 10,000 to 3 in 1000 |

**Table 2.10** Imaging studies: comparative radiation and cancer risk.

### Magnetic resonance imaging

Magnetic resonance imaging is good for visualising soft tissues, and it does not use radiation. MRI is also used to produce images of the effects of bone pathologies, for example in cases of infection and tumour.

**Principles**  An MRI scanner applies a strong magnetic field to an area of interest, causing hydrogen atoms to align parallel to the magnetic field and spin like a spinning top (i.e. precess). Electromagnetic radiation or a radiofrequency pulse is then applied to the precessing nuclei. When this is turned off, the nuclei return to their original precession around the external magnetic field. This involves two processes: T1 and T2 relaxation. The information is then converted into an image by computers in the MRI scanner.

**Terminology**  T1-weighted images convey the longitudinal relaxation time of tissues, whereas T2-weighted images depict the transverse relaxation time.

- Hyperintense tissue is brighter than adjacent tissue (e.g. water is hyperintense on T2-weighted images, and fat is hyperintense on T1-weighted images)
- Hypointense tissue is darker than adjacent tissue (e.g. water and fat are hypointense on T1-weighted images)

**Advantages**  Magnetic resonance imaging provides superb contrast between different soft tissues, and the resolution is higher than that of CT. There is no exposure to ionising radiation.

**Disadvantages**  Being in the MRI scanner can provoke claustrophobia in some patients. The examination time is longer than that of CT. MRI is contraindicated in patients with a pacemaker because the pacemaker heats up causing induction of ventricular fibrillation and damage to the pacemaker circuit. Some pacemakers are MR compatible, but the safest course of action is to assume all pacemakers are incompatible. Check with the scanning department if there is any doubt about contraindications for an MR scan.

## Ultrasound

For isolated structures such as the Achilles tendon or the patella tendon, ultrasound is a reliable and quick investigation.

**Principles** An ultrasound probe transmits high-frequency (1–15 MHz) pulses

> ### Clinical insight
>
> Magnetic resonance imaging is contraindicated in patients with:
> * some types of pacemaker
> * non-compatible aneurysm clips
> * cochlear implants
> * intraocular foreign body

of sound into the body. Some of the soundwaves reflect back, i.e. echo, to the probe and are detected by a transducer. The transducer calculates the distance between the probe and the echogenic tissue, based on the speed of sound in tissue (1540 m/s) and the time of return of each echo. The distance data are converted into two-dimensional greyscale images.

**Terminology** Structures are described in terms of their echogenicity.
* Anechoic structures do not produce any internal echoes
* Hypoechoic structures are less bright than adjacent areas
* Hyperechoic structures are brighter than adjacent areas

**Advantages** Ultrasound is safe and inexpensive. It is readily available for bedside use.

**Disadvantages** The technique is heavily operator-dependent. It is of limited use when examining bones and structures deep within the body, such as the retroperitoneum.

### Joint aspiration

Joint aspiration, i.e. arthrocentesis, is the removal of synovial fluid from a joint for analysis. It can be done with or without imaging guidance, and in or out of theatre (**Figure 2.4**). It is carried out for diagnostic reasons (e.g. in cases of arthritis), therapeutic reasons (e.g. to relieve discomfort) or both.

### Diagnostic aspiration

Diagnostic aspiration is indicated for any patient with an inflamed joint, and the results can help in the diagnosis of

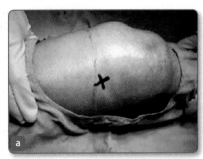

**Figure 2.4** Knee aspiration. (a) The point of aspiration is marked, and after injection of local anaesthetic, (b) a thick, bloody aspirate is drawn.

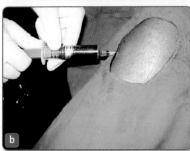

## Clinical insight

The knee is the easiest joint to aspirate, because it is close to the surface and generally produces a large effusion.

sepsis, gout, pseudogout and arthritis. Aspirate is sent for Gram staining; cell count; microscopy, sensitivities and cultures; and crystal analysis.

In cases of suspected septic arthritis, aspirate is immediately sent for Gram staining and culture and sensitivity testing. The results are essential to the diagnosis of infection, and also indicate suitable antibiotics. Aspiration and microbiological analysis must be carried out before antibiotics are prescribed.

### Therapeutic aspiration

Large effusions or haemarthroses can be very painful. The pain is temporarily relieved by therapeutic aspiration, although effusions often recollect.

## Blood tests

Blood tests are often the initial investigations when assessing a surgical patient. They may be diagnostic, allow an assessment of disease severity or indicate the patient's fitness for a surgical procedure.

Blood tests commonly carried out for surgical patients include full blood count, urea and electrolytes and a random glucose test (**Table 2.11**). These are mandatory for any patient who has bled as a result of injury, may have been or is dehydrated, has a chronic medical condition or is elderly.

No blood test is diagnostic. All have some degree of limitation of either sensitivity or specificity.

## Blood transfusion

All patients undergoing open surgery have a 'group and save', i.e. their blood group is determined and the blood is screened for the presence of common red cell antigens. If blood loss is anticipated or the patient has been bleeding, cross-matched blood must be ordered. In an emergency situation, give O negative blood because this is readily available. Type-specific blood takes time to obtain because the patient needs a test to

| Test | Relevance |
|------|-----------|
| Full blood count | Blood loss, presence of infection |
| Urea and electrolytes | Dehydration, hypovolaemia, adequacy of resuscitation |
| Clotting screen | Jaundice, clotting disorders, major haemorrhage |
| Group and save | Before anticipated blood loss or transfusion |
| Glucose measurement | Diabetes, loss of glycaemic control |

**Table 2.11** Common blood tests for orthopaedic patients.

determine their type, although fully-typed and antibody-tested (cross-matched) blood is the safest to give.

## Infection markers

Infection is indicated by increased white cell count along with markers of inflammation such as increased erythrocyte sedimentation rate and C-reactive protein. These markers are also used to monitor the response of infection to intervention.

Serum levels of certain antibiotics are also assayed to ensure that the levels of the antibiotic are within therapeutic range.

## Microbiology

Sepsis is a common complication of surgery. It varies from minor wound infection to life-threatening septic shock.

Appropriate microbiological specimens, for example blood, tissue fluid or pus, are collected and sent to the microbiology laboratory for analysis. Samples are taken before a patient is started on antibiotics. This increases the chances of identifying the causative organism and indicates suitable antibiotics.

## Specific disease markers

More specific markers in blood may be measured to help to monitor and/or diagnose orthopaedic disease, for example:

- in autoimmune conditions, rheumatoid factor in rheumatoid arthritis and antinuclear antibody panel in systemic lupus erythematosus
- tumour markers, for example monoclonal protein in multiple myeloma
- genetic testing, for example for Charcot–Marie–Tooth disease, muscular dystrophies, Prader–Willi syndrome

Nerve conduction studies and needle electromyography

Nerve conduction studies and needle electromyelography are used to evaluate peripheral nerve function. The former are used to confirm nerve entrapment syndromes such as carpal syndrome (see page 33).

In the setting of nerve injury, nerve conduction studies are used in conjunction with electromyelography to assess nerve and muscle injury and reinnervation.

## 2.4 Management

For traumatic presentations, the optimal outcome is restoration of the patient's preinjury level of function. In more chronic conditions, such as osteoarthritis, the aim is a pain-free functional return to activities of daily living, work and leisure. For arthritic joints, this usually requires joint fusion or replacement.

### Conservative management

Many orthopaedic disorders are best managed by not doing anything, for example asymptomatic ganglions, lipomas, hallux valgus and

> **Guiding principle**
>
> The aims of management always depend on the injury or disease AND the patient. Expectations of function are very subjective and should be clearly established with the patient.

many paediatric conditions. Reassurance and education are all that the patient requires in these cases. Other non-invasive programmes of rest, support and physical therapy successfully treat some orthopaedic conditions.

### Physiotherapy

Physiotherapy is used in management of the full range of orthopaedic complaints and improves patients' condition in several ways:

- muscle-strengthening regimes address joint problems and muscle imbalance
- improve range of motion at joints
- improve proprioception and joint conditioning

The physiotherapist takes a holistic view of the patient and, where necessary, will start with basic gait retraining, posture and flexibility. Manual therapies and massage are employed for specific problems.

### Medication

Drugs have a limited but important role in orthopaedic practice.

- Analgesics and anti-inflammatory agents help relieve pain and inflammation
- Long-acting drugs [e.g. disease-modifying agents of rheumatoid disease (DMARDs), methotrexate, infliximab]

are preferred in chronic disorders such as rheumatoid arthritis
- Short-acting drugs are preferred in acute infection and trauma
- Muscle relaxants (e.g. baclofen) are useful to relieve painful muscle spasms
- Antibiotics are extremely useful in acute and chronic infections of bones and joints; broad-spectrum agents are usually preferred
- Hormones used in orthopaedics include growth hormones for short stature, stilbestrol for metastatic carcinomas, anabolic steroids for growth failure and marrow stimulation, and oestrogens for osteoporosis
- Bisphosphonates for the secondary prevention of osteoporotic fractures
- Specific drugs include vitamin C for scurvy and vitamin D for rickets and osteomalacia
- Cytotoxic drugs are used as chemotherapeutic agents for malignant tumours (e.g. duxorubicin for soft tissue sarcoma)
- Drugs to prevent venous thromboembolisms, e.g low molecular weight heparin

## Antibiotics

Antibiotics have two main uses in orthopaedics: preoperative prophylaxis and treatment of infection. They are also given prophylactically to all patients with an open fracture. Local policy dictates which antibiotics are used in which circumstances. Most prophylaxis and treatment is targeted at skin commensals, i.e. *Staphylococcus* and *Streptococcus*.

Chronic osteomyelitis is difficult to treat. It is best managed in a specialist limb reconstruction centre with a multidisciplinary approach. Infected metalwork can necessitate long-term use of antibiotics or removal of the infected metalwork. Recovery can take months and often entails a lot of discomfort and inconvenience to the patient.

## Fracture management

**Table 2.12** lists questions to consider when managing fractures.

| Management question | Rationale |
|---|---|
| Is further information on the fracture needed, e.g. imaging studies? | Enough imaging information to decide on management, surgery, reduction? Need more on articular or fracture components? CT scan if yes? Need more to plan surgical approach and reduction, position of reduction hardware and/or devices? |
| Is the position of the fracture acceptable? | Fracture alignment acceptable without further reduction? In a child, what is the capacity for remodelling? |
| Is the fracture stable? | Will fracture displace if load supplied? Internal fix or plaster of Paris required for stability? |
| Does the fracture need reduction? | Need to reduce fracture to a satisfactory position? Angulated, shortened, and rotated fractures require reduction. Rules for acceptable deformity vary between according to bone fractured and fracture site |
| Does it need anatomical reduction? | Fractures around joints require anatomical reduction |
| How may reduction be achieved? | Reduction achieved by open or closed methods. Extra-articular and paediatric fractures use closed; complex fractures (e.g. articular) use open. Some reduction facilitated by minimally invasive approaches, or pins or K wires used to 'joystick' the fragments |
| How is the reduction held? | Strongest available implant chosen. Secure fixation allows early range of motion and weight bearing. Implants include screws, plates, anatomical plates, intramedullary devices, external fixation. A combination is sometimes used. Assess if structural and/or void-filling bone graft needed. |
| Is there any associated injury? | Nerve or blood vessel injuries, skin loss, associated soft tissue injuries may need repair (involve vascular/plastic surgeons). Other injuries away from fracture may require attention. Use multiple surgeons to attend to multiple injuries and reduce time in surgery? |

**Table 2.12** Questions in fracture management. *Continues opposite*

| Management question | Rationale |
|---|---|
| What is the timing of intervention? | Open, limb-threatening injuries and dislocations require immediate attention. Other injuries may benefit from a pre-surgery delay to allow soft tissues to settle, provided fracture is splinted. Patient may have other injuries requiring management prior to fracture |
| Will the patient tolerate the treatment? | Patients need to be informed; not all want surgery. Make patients aware of postoperative, plan including non-weight bearing status and compliance with regimes. Alternate options are sought if patient not likely to comply |
| What are the potential complications of the planned intervention? | Inform patient of risks and benefits: including not having treatment. There are risks to nerves and blood vessels, and of infection. Give the likelihood of metalwork being removed or requirements for other procedures. Immobilising patients increases the DVT risk |

**Table 2.12** *Continued*

## Clinical insight

A stable fracture:

- does not displace under physiological load
- requires no treatment other than analgesia
- may require splinting to treat pain
- allows early movement (e.g. walking), which prevents long-term stiffness and functional deficit

### Reduction and stabilisation

Fracture reduction means correcting any displacement present. The anatomy is then stabilised with a back slab or plaster of Paris cast or fixed internally with screws and plates, or externally with pins and an external frame. This provides a secure environment for healing. Reduction may require incision (open reduction) or is carried out closed.

The following abbreviations are used to describe the method of reduction and stabilisation.

- CRIF: closed reduction and internal fixation
- ORIF: open reduction and internal fixation

- CREF: closed reduction external fixation
- OREF: open reduction external fixation

**Timing of intervention** Determining when to treat depends on the injury and any associated conditions. Situations requiring urgent intervention include cases of:

- dislocation
- open fracture
- pulseless limb
- compartment syndrome

Closed, relatively uncomplicated injuries are managed on an urgent but scheduled basis. This allows optimisation of treatment by the best available operative team during a scheduled operating list.

Prioritisation is case by case. For example, fixation of a fracture to the proximal femur in an elderly patient is completed within 24 h of admission, whereas fixation of a calcaneal fracture in a younger patient may be delayed by 2 weeks to allow soft tissue swelling to settle. The elderly patient benefits from early intervention, which allows early stable, pain-free mobilisation and prevents medical deterioration. For the younger patient, a better outcome is achieved by allowing the contusion and swelling to settle, resulting in a lower likelihood of postoperative wound complication.

**Anatomical reduction** Restoration of normal anatomy is the goal of fracture reduction. It is particularly important in fractures near or involving joint surfaces, because it has a greater effect on functional outcome. Intrartricular fractures are anatomically reduced and fixed to be as stable as possible, to facilitate early range of motion. This is not always possible, particularly if there is significant comminution, crushing of the fragments or gross damage to the articular cartilage.

## Devices

The main devices used in orthopaedics are:

- plaster of Paris
- Kirschner wires
- plates and screws

- intramedullary nails
- external fixators with wires and/or half-pins

**Plaster of Paris**  A plaster of Paris cast increases stability either temporarily or as part of non-operative management of a fracture or soft tissue injury.

The first step in fracture management is application of a back slab. This is mandatory in the first aid treatment of any fracture. A back slab is a cast that encircles about 60–70% of the limb, splinting the limb but allowing for further swelling. In the case of an acute injury with ongoing initial swelling, a full cast may become too tight, which could lead to compartment syndrome or a related complication.

Plaster of Paris is used to immobilise either stable fractures that require reduction or minimally-displaced fractures.

Local anaesthetic agents must not be used with adrenaline (epinephrine) in digits. This may cause irreversible ischemia as a consequence of arterial constriction. Local anaesthetic has a maximum safe dosage. This dosage varies depending on the agent.

**The Thomas splint**  The Thomas splint is a device used to treat femoral shaft fractures. It definitively treats paediatric fractures and temporary-splints adult fractures. It consists of a metal frame with a padded ring at the proximal end. The ring rests on the pelvis; skin traction is applied and tied to the distal aspect of the splint. This is tensioned to provide counter-traction.

**Principles**  The patient should be supine. The splint is sized for length and proximal ring circumference: 4 cm are added to the circumference to allow for swelling and 20 cm added to the length to attain the length of the splint. Adhesive skin traction is applied to the leg and secured to the leg with a crepe bandage.

The Thomas splint is then applied to the leg. The splint is pre-prepared with a sling to support the leg. Traction is applied distally and the cords of the skin traction are secured to the distal aspect of the splint. The limb is elevated by tilting the bed and a counterweight of approximately 5–8 kg is applied.

After applying the splint bandage circumferentially to the leg, check regularly for any pressure points between the thigh and the proximal ring. Perform anteroposterior and lateral radiographs of the femur to confirm position.

## Local anaesthetic

Local anaesthetic is used to produce a haematoma block to enable pain-free reduction of, for example a wrist fracture. Sufficient analgesia is achieved by infiltration of the anaesthetic into the fracture haematoma. Many wounds are explored under local anaesthesia.

> ### Clinical insight
>
> Always check the patient's allergy status before giving the first dose of an antibiotic. Anaphylaxis is uncommon but potentially life-threatening. If the patient is allergic to a particular antibiotic, give the unit's alternative antibiotic to prevent harmful complications.

## Surgery

Surgery is considered when all other treatment options have been exhausted. It should not worsen the condition of the patient.

## Osteotomy

An osteotomy is the creation of a surgical fracture. It used, for example, to:
- correct excessive angulations, bowing or rotation of a long bone
- compensate for and correct malalignment of a joint
- correct leg length inequality by shortening or lengthening
- alter the line of weight-bearing and increase hip stability (e.g. abduction osteotomy)
- relieve pain in an arthritic hip (e.g. in displacement osteotomy) or knee (e.g. in high tibial osteotomy)

## Arthrodesis

Arthrodesis is the fusion of joints, which increases stability but reduces mobility. Because it limits joint function, arthroplasty is more common in the hip and knee. However, arthrodesis can be used for:
- gross destruction of the joints, as in rheumatoid arthritis, Charcot's joints or advanced osteoarthritis

- quiescent tubercular arthritis
- gross instability as a result of muscle paralysis, for example in poliomyelitis
- permanent correction of a deformity

Arthrodesis involves gaining access to the joint either arthroscopically or as an open procedure. Joint surfaces are prepared by denuding the joint of the articular cartilage with exposure of cancellous bone. The joint is fixed in its permanent position with compression across the joint surfaces. The compression/fixation is achieved with a combination of screws and or plates. Bone grafts are used for both structural reasons and to stimulate bony union.

> ## Clinical insight
>
> Arthrodesis (joint fusion) is done in the most functional position. For example, the knee is fused at 20° flexion, and the shoulder at 30° abduction, 30° flexion and 30° internal rotation.

### Arthroplasty

Arthroplasty is the construction of a new mobile joint. Indications include:

- advanced hip, knee, shoulder, elbow, hand and foot arthritis
- quiescent destructive tuberculous arthritis of hip and elbow
- mal- or non-union of a fracture of the femoral neck
- primary treatment of a fracture considered unreconstructable, e.g. knee replacement for a comminuted tibial plateau fracture, hip replacement for primary treatment of an intra-articular proximal femoral fracture
- correction of a deformity (rare), for example hallux valgus

There are three types of arthroplasty.

- In excision arthroplasty (e.g. of the hip, elbow or metatarsophalangeal joint), one or both articular surfaces are excised; the gap eventually fills with fibrous tissue, allowing some mobility
- In hemireplacement arthroplasty, one articulating surface is replaced with a prosthesis, e.g. cemented Thompson's hemiarthroplasty for a displaced intracapsular neck of femur fracture
- In total replacement arthroplasty (e.g. total hip or knee replacement for osteoarthritis or rheumatoid arthritis), both

articular surfaces are replaced. Stems are usually made of metal, although in hip arthroplasty the cup is ceramic or polyethylene. Implants are specifically designed to be cemented or uncemented

## Bone grafting

Bone grafts provide a scaffold for new bone growth, and are used, for example:

- to promote union in cases of non-union fractures
- for intra-articular or extraarticular fusion in arthrodesis
- to fill a defect or cavity in a bone

The bone used comes from the patient (in an autograft), another living person (in an allograft), a cadaver or an animal (a xenograft). Alternatively, artificial bone made of hydroxyapatite is used. Cancellous bone is usually taken from the iliac crest, and cortical bone from the fibula.

## Tendon surgeries

Tendon surgeries are either tendon transfers or tendon grafts.

> **Clinical insight**
>
> Cadaveric bone is either fresh-frozen, freeze-dried or demineralised.

- In tendon transfers, a healthy muscle insertion is moved to a new site to fulfill function; this procedure is used in cases of muscle paralysis (e.g. peripheral motor neuropathy), muscle imbalance (cerebral palsy) or rupture
- In tendon grafts, a graft (e.g. from a toe extensor) is used to bridge a gap; this procedure is used in reconstructive hand surgery

## Equalisation of leg length

This is done by lengthening one leg or shortening the other, or in children, by arrest of epiphyseal growth (e.g. arthrogryposis).

## Tumour excision

This is the main treatment for most bone cancers. Amputation may be required, but limb salvage surgery, which is possible in 90% of limb bone cancers, can be carried out to leave a functional limb. Removed bone is replaced with an endoprosthesis, for example one made of a cobalt–chrome–molybdenum alloy.

## Amputation

Amputation is considered if a limb is severely damaged or if there is extensive neurovascular damage causing ischaemia. A functioning joint is left, if possible, but amputation must extend as proximally as necessary, given the clinical findings. Initially, it may be necessary to carry out an extensive debridement, with formal stump fashioning at a later date.

Indications for amputation include chronic resistant infection, severe trauma, neoplasm, and deformity. Most tertiary centres have an amputation care team who deal with preoperative counselling and planning, as well as continuing postoperative care and physiotherapy.

# Spine

The spine provides structural support for the body and protection for the spinal cord and nerves, and allows a degree of mobility in several planes. At each vertebral level, paired spinal nerves exit the central nervous system; at this point they are especially vulnerable to compression. Furthermore, the dynamic, stress-bearing nature of the back and spine means that it is a common site of pain resulting from mechanical or neural injury.

## 3.1 Clinical scenario

### Back pain

### Background

A 58-year-old woman has had intermittent back pain over the past few years. While looking after her young grandson at the weekend, she tried to lift him but had sudden, severe lower lumbar back pain and could hardly move afterwards. Since then, she had been resting at home and taking painkillers. However, the pain has worsened, and she has had some weakness and numbness in her right foot as well as difficulty passing urine, so she has presented at the emergency department.

### History

The patient has a past medical history of hypertension and long-standing back pain, for which she takes co-codamol as required. She lives with her husband; they are both retired but live independently, and her medical conditions do not limit her activities of daily living. She does not require walking aids.

### Examination

Inspection finds normal alignment and no deformity. The pain means that the patient has difficulty walking. She has tenderness over her lower lumbar spine, and because of the pain is unable to fully flex or extend her back. On neurological examination, she has normal tone in both lower limbs.

The straight leg raise test gives a positive result on the right. Power is decreased on the right in ankle dorsiflexion and the long toe extensors. Sensation is decreased on the dorsum of the foot and the medial malleolus. An ankle reflex cannot be elicited, and the results of plantar reflex testing are equivocal.

On rectal examination, anal tone is decreased. A bladder scan confirms that the patient has urinary retention.

### Differential diagnosis
Possible causes of the patient's symptoms and signs are:
- cauda equina syndrome
- conus medullaris infarction
- prolapsed vertebral disc
- spinal stenosis
- vascular claudication
- exacerbation of chronic degenerative disc disease
- musculoskeletal back pain

Given the abnormal neurology and urinary retention, cauda equina syndrome is the most likely diagnosis.

### Investigations
An urgent MRI scan is requested to confirm any nerve root compression and its cause, including disc pathology, tumour or infection.

> **Clinical insight**
>
> The straight leg raise test confirms irritation of the lumbar nerve root when pain is elicited in the affected leg by passive elevation (usually by 30–60°) with the knee extended. Lower the leg until the pain passes. Passively dorsiflex the ankle. If the pain is reproduced, this is Lasègue's sign.

## 3.2 Anatomy

The spine comprises 33 vertebrae and associated ligaments, fibrocartilaginous intervertebral discs and facet joints. It is divided into five regions (**Figure 3.1**):
- the cervical region (7 vertebrae)
- the thoracic region (12 vertebrae)
- the lumbar region (5 vertebrae)
- the sacrum (5 fused vertebrae)
- the coccyx (4 fused vertebrae)

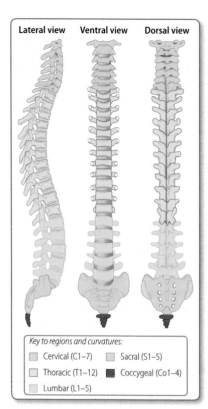

Lateral view    Ventral view    Dorsal view

**Figure 3.1** Regions of the spine.

*Key to regions and curvatures:*
- ☐ Cervical (C1–7)    ☐ Sacral (S1–5)
- ☐ Thoracic (T1–12)   ☐ Coccygeal (Co1–4)
- ☐ Lumbar (L1–5)

The normal spine is curved in the sagittal plane. The cervical and lumbar regions curve anteriorly (lordosis), and the thoracic and sacral regions curve posteriorly (kyphosis).

## Spinal columns

The spine is described in terms of three columns: anterior, middle and posterior.

The anterior column comprises:
- the anterior longitudinal ligament
- the anterior annular ligament
- the anterior half of the vertebral body

The middle column consists of:
- the posterior longitudinal ligament
- the posterior annular ligament
- the posterior half of the vertebral body

The posterior column comprises:
- the pedicles
- the spinous process
- the posterior ligaments
- the neural arch

## Vertebrae

Individual vertebrae consist of an anterior part, the vertebral body, and a posterior part, the vertebral arch. The vertebral arch is made up of pedicles, laminae, transverse processes and a spinous process (**Figure 3.2**). The vertebral body and vertebral arch form the vertebral foramen.

Vertebrae differ in shape and size at various levels. For example, all 12 thoracic vertebrae have demifacets that articulate with the corresponding ribs, and their spinous processes are long and slope downwards, and lumbar vertebrae have large, strong vertebral bodies.

## Intervertebral discs

Intervertebral discs form fibrocartilaginous joints between adjacent vertebral bodies. Each disc comprises a jelly-like inner

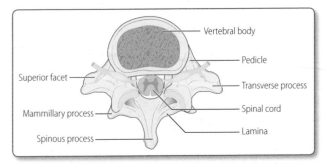

**Figure 3.2** Cross-section of the spine.

nucleus pulposus and an outer fibrous ring called the annulus fibrosus. The disc acts as a shock absorber and also distributes pressure evenly to adjacent vertebrae under a compressive force. Superior and inferior facet joints on each vertebra increase stability and restrict movement.

## Ligaments

Ligaments pass between the spinous processes and laminae of adjacent vertebrae (**Figure 3.3**). Two adjacent vertebral discs and their associated ligamentous structures form a functional spinal unit called a motion segment.

## Spinal cord

The spinal cord passes through the spinal canal, the space formed by successive vertebral foramina. It is the main pathway connecting the brain to the peripheral nervous system. It transmits motor signals from, and conveys sensory information to the brain. It also contains the neural circuits responsible for reflexes, i.e. actions that occur independently of the brain. The spinal cord contains white matter peripherally and grey

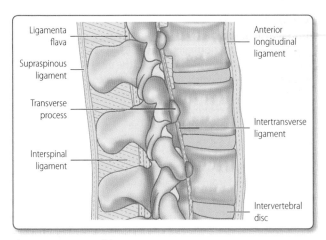

**Figure 3.3** Ligaments of the spine.

matter medially (**Figure 3.4**). The white matter is neural tracts of sensory and motor neurones. The grey matter is neuronal cell bodies in a butterfly-shape around the central canal.

## Meninges

The spinal cord and spinal nerve roots are covered by meninges within the spinal canal and intervertebral foramina. From superficial to deep, they are:
- the epidural space
- the dura mater
- the subdural space
- the arachnoid mater
- the subarachnoid space
- the pia mater

## Levels of the spinal cord

The adult spinal cord extends from the foramen magnum and terminates as the medullary cone (conus medullaris) at vertebral level L1–L2 (**Figure 3.5**). The anterior and posterior nerve roots at each spinal level join one another and exit the intervertebral foramina, forming spinal nerves from C1 to S5; they are mixed sensory and motor. C1–C7 exit above the associated vertebrae, C8 exits below the C7 vertebrae and T1–S5 exit below their respective vertebrae.

The spinal cord normally ends at L1, so lower nerve roots course some distance before exiting the intervertebral foramina. This is relevant when considering the consequences of a spinal cord injury at a given level. The lower spinal nerves form the cauda equina (Latin, 'horse's tail'). The cauda equina ends at S2, with termination of the dural sac.

## Sensory and motor tracts

Neural tracts ascend and descend the spinal cord, carrying neural signals to and from the brain. Generally, descending tracts carry motor information and ascending tracts carry sensory information (**Figure 3.4**).

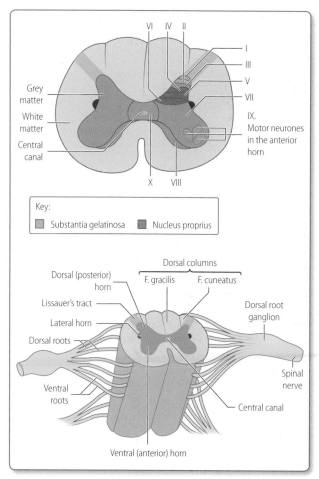

**Figure 3.4** Internal anatomy of the spinal cord. The grey matter comprises three 'horns': the dorsal (posterior) horn carrying sensory fibres, the ventral (anterior) horn carrying motor fibres and the lateral horn carrying fibres of the sympathetic division of the autonomic nervous system; the grey matter is divided into laminae I–X.

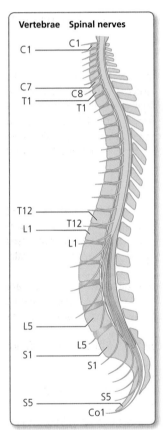

**Figure 3.5** Levels of the spinal cord.

Sensory information is carried by sensory peripheral nerves. Each of these nerves is a projection of a neurone with a cell body in one of the dorsal root ganglia, clusters of neuronal cell bodies outside the spinal cord. These neurones synapse in the cord, decussate and ascend, synapsing again in the thalamus before terminating in the sensory cortex.

Motor neurones also decussate in the spinal cord. Their cell bodies are contained within the ventral grey matter of the cord. Peripheral nerves project from these neurones to innervate muscle on the side of the body contralateral to the cortex initiating the signal.

## Vascular supply

The spinal cord is supplied by three arteries that run along its length: the anterior spinal artery and the right and left posterior spinal arteries. These arise in the brain from the intracranial part of the vertebral artery. They are reinforced serially by the spinal branches from the ascending cervical artery, the cervical part of the vertebral artery, the posterior intercostal arteries and the lumbar arteries.

## Surface anatomy

Several features of the spine can be palpated via the skin and are useful anatomical landmarks in examinations and procedures (**Figures 3.6 and 3.7**). The tips of the spinous processes are palpable within the midline groove of the back, especially during flexion.

The spinous processes and the spaces between them are used to mark the levels of underlying structures or planes and thereby help guide procedures for spinal anaesthesia. For example:

- C7 is the most prominent spinous process on the inferior neck
- T12 is at the medial end of the 12th rib
- L2 marks the inferior limit of the spinal cord in adults
- L4 marks the highest point of the iliac crest

Transverse processes mark the positions of spinal nerves. Therefore they are useful landmarks during procedures such as regional nerve or plexus anaesthesia.

---

# 3.3 Examination

## Key signs

Key signs to assess for include gait abnormality, deformity, tenderness and abnormal neurology.

## Examination sequence

Examination follows a system of 'look, feel and move' and a thorough neurological examination of the upper and lower limbs.

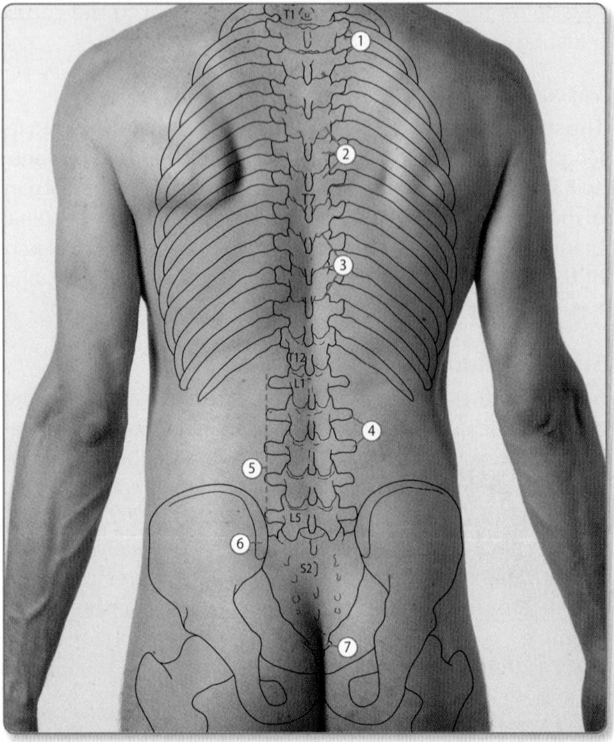

**Figure 3.6** Posterior view of the vertebra and intervertebral joints. ① Costotransverse joints, ② vertebral laminae, ③ facet/zygapophyseal joints, ④ transverse processes, ⑤ vertical plane aligned with the posterior superior iliac spine landmarks the lumbar vertebral transverse processes, ⑥ posterior superior iliac spine, ⑦ sacrococcygeal joint.

## Look

- Observe the overall alignment
- Is the patient's posture balanced?
- Assess the curvature of the spine; is it normal? Is there evidence of scoliosis or kyphosis?
- Are there any scars indicating previous spinal surgery?

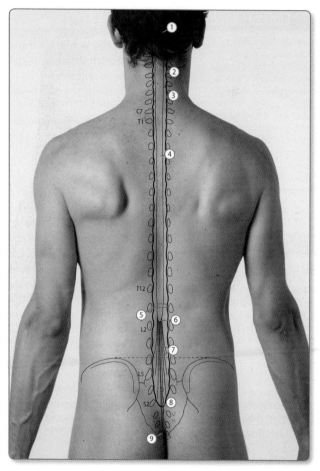

**Figure 3.7** Meninges, spinal cord and spinal nerves within the vertebral canal (cutaway view). ① Foramen magnum, ② dura mater lined internally with arachnoid mater, ③ subarachnoid space filled with cerebrospinal fluid, ④ spinal cord covered in pia mater, ⑤ vertebral canal containing spinal cord and nerves within meningeal coverings, ⑥ conus medullaris (termination of spinal cord), ⑦ cauda equina, ⑧ termination of subarachnoid space, ⑨ sacral hiatus.

## Clinical insight

After spinal trauma patients are immobilised and thoroughly examined. They are fully exposed to assess for abrasions, bruising or wounds, then 'logrolled' (manoeuvred without moving the spinal column) to assess for bruising, abrasions, spinal tenderness and deformity, and to perform a rectal examination. A neurological examination is performed and a sensory examination completed to determine whether the injury is in the anterior or dorsal column.

## Clinical insight

The bulbocavernosus reflex is always checked; it is contraction of the anal sphincter in response to stimulation of the trigone of the bladder. This is done with a squeeze on the glans of the penis, a tap on the mons pubis or a pull on a urethral catheter. Absence of this reflex indicates spinal shock.

### Feel

- Palpate along the length of the spine for bony tenderness over the spinous processes
- Palpate the sacroiliac joints
- Is there any muscular tenderness paraspinally?

### Move

- Check movements of the cervical spine by asking the patient to flex and extend forwards and backwards, flex laterally and rotate (**Figure 3.8**)
- Check rotation of the thoracic spine (**Figure 3.9**)
- Ask the patient to flex and extend the lumbar spine; do they have pain or limited movement?
- Check lateral bend by asking the patient to run their hand down the outside of each leg
- Check rotation of lumbar spine

### Function

- Is the patient's gait normal? Do they lean forwards (indicating spinal stenosis) or have a wide-based gait (indicating myelopathy)?
- Conduct a full neurological examination of the upper and lower limbs; test motor and sensory responses and reflexes; and carry out rectal examination (see page 36)

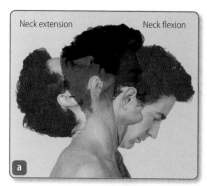

**Figure 3.8** Neck movements: (a) Extension (60°) flexion (50°). (b) Lateral flexion (45°).

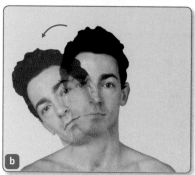

# 3.4 Cauda equina syndrome

Cauda equina syndrome is a mixture of symptoms caused by spinal nerve root compression as a result of disc herniation. It is an emergency because it leads to irreversible neurological damage.

### Epidemiology

Cauda equina syndrome is an uncommon condition that usually, but not always, presents without a history of trauma. Atraumatic cauda equina syndrome occurs primarily in older patients (age > 50 years). Traumatic cauda equina syndrome occurs at any age.

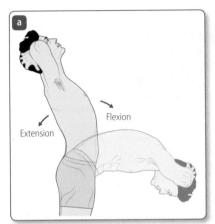

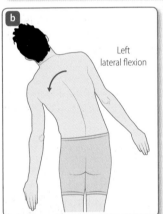

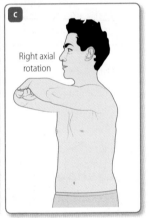

**Figure 3.9** Spine movements. (a) Extension/flexion, (b) left lateral flexion, (c) right axial rotation.

## Causes

The syndrome is caused by multilevel lumbosacral root compression within the lumbar spinal canal. The most common cause is disc herniation. Other causes include spinal tumours (including metastases), epidural haematoma or abscesses and spinal trauma.

## Clinical features

The patient often has a mix of symptoms, including:
- back pain and radicular pain (a sharp pain that projects in a dermatomal distribution)
- lower limb sensorimotor symptoms
- bowel and bladder dysfunction
- saddle anaesthesia (numbnness in the inner thigh, perineum and buttocks)

On examination, the patients are in pain and often complain of lower back tenderness. The straight leg raise test is often positive, often bilaterally. The patient occasionally has reduced power in muscles supplied by affected roots, with decreased or absent reflexes (lower motor neurone symptoms). Patients usually describe numbness in specific dermatomes and in the saddle region.

Urinary retention may be present, but it is often a late sign and indicates a poorer prognosis. Bowel disturbances include incontinence, constipation and loss of anal tone.

## Investigations

Plain radiographs are unlikely to be helpful. MRI is the gold standard (**Figure 3.10**), but if it is contraindicated a CT is done.

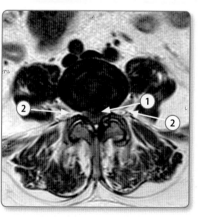

**Figure 3.10** MRI scan showing central disc prolapse ① compressing the exiting nerve roots ② in cauda equina syndrome.

The bladder is scanned to check for urinary retention. If the cause of cauda equina syndrome is unknown, blood tests are used to look for signs of an infection or inflammation. They include full blood count, urea and electrolytes, C-reactive protein, erythrocyte sedimentation rate and bone profile. Electromyography often shows evidence of denervation.

## Management

Urgent surgical decompression is required. The patient is usually transferred to the nearest spinal unit. A pre- and post-void bladder scan is carried out, and a catheter inserted. Appropriate analgesia is provided. After surgery, intensive rehabilitation and physical therapy are required.

**Complications** The risk of complications increases with the length of time that passes before the patient is taken to theatre. Better outcomes are achieved if surgery is carried out within 48 h of presentation. Complications include:

- bowel and bladder dysfunction
- erectile dysfunction
- motor weakness
- sensory disturbance
- disability due to a neurological deficit
- deep vein thrombosis or pulmonary embolism

# 3.5 Spinal fractures

Fractures occur at any point in the spine. Multiple bony levels may be involved, and the fracture may be contiguous or non-contiguous. The fracture may be associated with subluxation or dislocation.

The spinal cord or spinal nerves may be injured as a consequence of the fracture. The overriding principle in the management of spinal fractures is to prevent neurological injuries or further damage to the injured neurological structures.

## Fractures of the thoracic and lumbar vertebrae

Wedge fractures are typically caused by a fall; they are generally low-energy injuries occurring in osteoporotic bone. Burst fractures are usually caused by axial loading.

Chance fractures are flexion distraction fractures that occur when the spine is flexed around a pivot. They are often described as seatbelt fractures, because the thoracolumbar spine is subjected to forced flexion over a fixed point, such as the part of the seatbelt that crosses the lap. These injuries may have a large soft tissue or ligamentous component causing significant instability, so they may appear benign despite being grossly unstable.

Fracture dislocations usually occur as a consequence of high-energy trauma. They are, by definition, unstable.

Single-column injuries are generally stable. Fractures involving the middle column and either or both of the anterior or posterior columns must be considered unstable.

## Wedge fractures

**Figure 3.11** shows a wedge fracture of the lumbar vertebrae. This involves only the anterior column, so is usually considered stable.

The usual management is analgesia, use of a thoracolumbosacral orthosis brace and physiotherapy. The aim of treatment is to maintain extension at the lumbar spine and prevent kyphotic deformity at the level of the wedge.

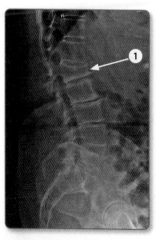

**Figure 3.11** Plain lateral radiograph of the lumbar spine, showing a wedge fracture of L1 ①.

### Burst fractures

**Figure 3.12** shows burst fractures of L1 and L2. **Figure 3.13** shows the extent of the L1 fracture and the involvement of all three columns. Burst fracture is usually a high-energy injury involving more than one column. As such, it is considered unstable.

A burst fracture configuration occasionally causes fragments of bone to encroach into the spinal canal. These retropulsed fragments of bone can compromise neural structures and therefore require surgical removal.

### Chance fractures

A Chance fracture occurs usually with rapid deceleration. Often, a seatbelt acts a pivot about which the flexion occurs. The spine fails under severe distraction or tension, causing failure of all three columns. The injury may be entirely confined to the soft tissues or through bone, or a combination of the two.

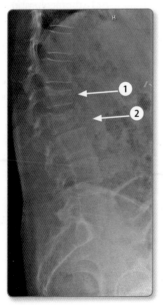

**Figure 3.12** Lateral radiograph of the lumbar spine, showing burst fractures of L1 ① and L2 ②.

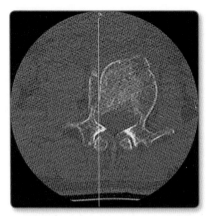

**Figure 3.13** Axial CT scan of the L1 vertebra, showing a burst fracture involving all three columns.

These injuries are markedly unstable. The paucity of radiological findings belies the extensive nature of this injury pattern.

### Clinical insight

Patients with fracture dislocation tend to have very unstable fractures. Therefore they are particularly vulnerable to the effects of rotation; logrolling must be carried out with the utmost care.

### Fracture dislocations

A fracture dislocation occurs when all three columns are involved, with loss of the normal relationships of the vertebrae. By definition, there is failure of the ligamentous constraints.

These injuries are markedly unstable. This injury pattern usually occurs as a consequence of significant trauma, such as that sustained in a road traffic accident or fall from a height.

### Cervical spine injuries

Cervical spine injuries consist of facet joint dislocations, subluxations, fractures and soft tissue injuries.

### Flexion injuries

Flexion injuries are generally caused by injuries causing flexion of the head on the neck, such as blows to the back of the head, falls and sports injuries. This type of injury usually causes an anterior wedge fracture pattern, which is generally stable.

## Flexion-with-rotation injuries

Flexion-with-rotation injuries usually give rise to a unifacetal dislocation. This appears on a lateral radiograph of the cervical spine as one vertebral body overlapping another by about a third. A complete facet joint dislocation is occasionally evident on the lateral radiograph as a vertebral body overlap of greater than one third. Both unifacetal and bifacetal dislocations occur with or without fracture.

## Extension injuries

Extension injuries are commonly caused by road traffic accidents, blows to the front of the head and sports injuries. They are often associated with an unstable injury. The anterior longitudinal ligament is ruptured. The injury is propagated through the intervertebral disc. The neck flexes forwards, back into position, after the initial force is removed. The only clue to the injury may be a small avulsion fracture at the anterior body of the vertebra.

These injuries are much like seatbelt injuries of the lumbar spine, except that the pivot is the posterior structures rather than the anterior ones. The benign radiographic appearance of extension injuries belies their potentially significantly unstable nature. Patients usually present with neurological signs at more than one level, because of the diffuse nature of the cord injury in hyperextension.

## Compression injuries

Compression injuries are sustained by application of an axial load. They commonly occur in diving injuries, injury from objects falling on to the head and sports injuries. They are the analogue of the burst fracture of the thoracolumbar spine and must be considered unstable. Retropulsed fragments may need to be removed surgically.

## C1 (atlas) fractures

These usually occur as a consequence of axial compression. They may be considered a burst type of injury. The ring of the atlas is usually fractured in four places, causing separation of the lateral masses. With flexion the transverse ligament, which restrains the odontoid peg, may rupture.

C1 fractures are particularly unstable. All patients with this type of fracture are at high risk of neurological compromise. **Figure 3.14** shows a fracture through the arch of C1.

## C2 fractures

The C2 vertebrae is called the axis and interlocks with C1, the atlas. The axis has a prominent bony spike, the odontoid peg, which allows the atlas to pivot and rotate. Fractures of the odontoid peg occur as a consequence of severe flexion or extension. These fractures are classified as type 1, 2 or 3 (**Figure 3.15**).

- Type 1 occurs at the tip of the peg
- Type 2 occurs at the junction of the body and the peg
- Type 3 involves the body of the vertebra (**Figure 3.16**)

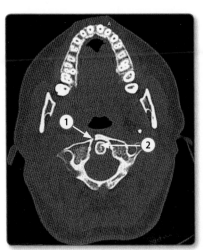

**Figure 3.14** Axial CT scan showing fracture at the arch of C1 (the atlas) ①. The odontoid peg is visible ②.

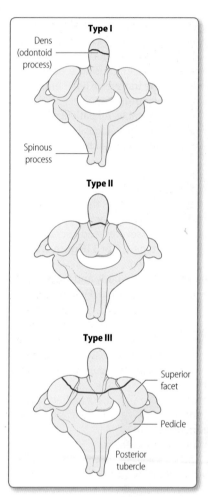

**Figure 3.15** Classification of odontoid peg fractures.

These injuries are potentially unstable and may cause significant neurological compromise, because they allow C2 and the distal vertebrae to sublux or translate around the peg fracture, which remains attached to C1 by the transverse ligament.

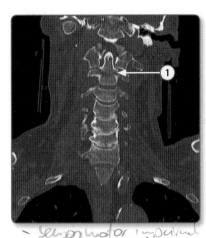

**Figure 3.16** Coronal CT scan showing a type 3 fracture of the odontoid peg ①.

## Management

Immediate management of all spinal injuries must consist of triple immobilisation and a primary survey in accordance with the Advanced Trauma Life Support protocol. Spinal palpation is are carried out, using logroll technique to move the patient (see page 345). If there is tenderness, neurological symptoms or signs, or both, a CT scan is obtained, if available. If CT is unavailable, anteroposterior and lateral radiographs are used.

Patients with suspected or confirmed spinal fractures are transferred to the regional spinal centre, or their case is at least discussed with staff from the centre.

Surgery for thoracolumbar spinal fractures is carried out to stabilise significantly unstable injuries, to remove any retropulsed fragments and to limit neurological compromise. Many injuries, particularly wedge fractures, are managed non-operatively with appropriate bracing.

Similar treatment principles apply to the management of cervical spine injuries. Many injuries are managed non-operatively with application of halo traction. Facetal dislocation is usually managed initially by traction to reduce the dislocation.

## 3.6 Spinal cord injury

Spinal cord injuries can either be temporary or permanent. They cause a range of neurological deficits: either motor, sensory or both.

Spinal cord injuries are divided into:
- complete injury, in which there is no motor or sensory function below the affected level
- incomplete injury, in which some motor or sensory function is spared below the affected level

### Epidemiology

Around 1200 patients in the UK are paralysed every year by a spinal cord injury. Just under half of these cases are caused by falls and 37% by road traffic accidents.

Spinal cord injuries occur in a bimodal distribution. Injuries in the young are associated with significant trauma, and in older patients with low-impact trauma and concurrent degenerative spinal changes.

### Causes

Spinal cord injuries have a primary or secondary cause.
- The primary cause is direct trauma; the effects of a spinal cord injury with a primary cause are often irreversible
- Secondary causes are associated with the injury sustained by the local soft tissues; spinal cord injuries with a secondary cause tend to evolve over time and relate to swelling resulting from an inflammatory response or bleeding into the soft tissues

Poor initial management of spinal trauma may lead to secondary injury. Such injuries are occasionally improved with the use of steroids. Advice from a tertiary centre on the management of spinal cord injuries must always be sought.

Neurological symptoms may present in neurogenic shock and in spinal shock (see page 83).

### Guiding principle

Up to 25% of spinal cord injuries are a result of improper spinal immobilisation and patient transport.

## Clinical features

Motor and sensory weakness or loss of function will occur below the level of the spinal cord injury. Regular assessment and documentation of neurological status is essential, because improvement or progression occasionally occur.

An American Spinal Injury Association impairment scale assessment is completed, rectal examination is carried out and the level of neurological injury is ascertained.

## Investigations

Urgent imaging, CT and then MRI are key to identifying the level and extent of the injury. The results also enable a management plan to be put in place as soon as possible. If surgery is likely to be required, blood samples are sent for urgent tests, including crossmatching.

## Management

A primary survey, including triple immobilisation, is immediately carried out. A patient with a high cervical injury occasionally require intubation as a matter of urgency, because of the potential loss of function of the muscles of respiration. The phrenic nerve with a root value of C3, C4 or C5 may be injured, which would also compromise respiration significantly.

Management varies greatly, depending on the condition of the patient and the level and classification of the injury. To prevent evolution of the injury, patients must be logrolled carefully for the purposes of examination. Management requires an extensive multidisciplinary team approach and a long-term programme of rehabilitation.

**Conservative management** Steroids are occasionally used to reduce local inflammation and swelling. The use of steroids depends on local protocols. Braces are frequently used to protect the injured tissue.

**Surgical management** This consists of stabilisation and decompression. Surgery is indicated when the neurological level is worsening or if spinal stability is needed to optimise the potential for rehabilitation.

**Complications**  Potential complications of spinal cord injuries include:

- autonomic dysfunction from disruption of the sympathetic pathway
- pulmonary embolism or deep vein thrombosis
- skin problems, e.g. pressure sores, caused by immobility
- bladder and bowel problems, e.g. recurrent infections resulting from incontinence or stasis

It is likely that the regional spinal centre will be responsible for the treatment of any patient with spinal cord injury, both acutely and in the long term.

## 3.7 Spinal metastases

Cancers that commonly metastasise to the bone are lung, prostate, thyroid, breast and renal cancer, and multiple myeloma. It is important to determine if a bony lesion is a metastasis or a primary bone tumour, or if it has another cause, because this dictates the investigations required and treatment given. Common sites for metastatic bone disease are the spine (50%), ribs, femur and pelvis.

### Clinical features

Spinal metastases present with ongoing pain, night pain and symptoms associated with the primary cause, for example weight loss and haematuria in cases of renal cell carcinoma. Pathological fractures (**Figure 3.17**) and cord compression result in a neurological deficit from the affected level.

### Investigations

The investigations required depend on the stage of diagnosis. If the patient is young with an unknown primary, blood tests, site-specific imaging (MRI or ultrasound) and a staging CT are needed. Osteolytic lesions are most commonly visible on radiography (**Figure 3.18**). Vertebral destruction is apparent on the anteroposterior radiograph as the loss of normal radiological architecture. The pedicle, which appears as a circle on anteroposterior views, is often lost (**Figures 3.19**). If the patient has advanced cancer, there may be no need for further investigations.

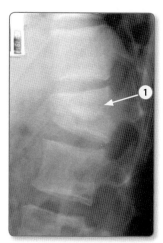

**Figure 3.17** Lateral lumbar spine radiograph showing a pathological wedge fracture of L2 (1).

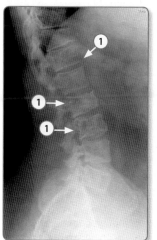

**Figure 3.18** Lateral spine radiograph showing lytic lesions (1) of the lumbar vertebrae.

MRI is needed If there is spinal cord involvement. It is a highly sensitive investigation in the diagnosis of tumour in cases in which there is any doubt (**Figure 3.20**).

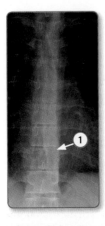
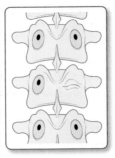

**Figure 3.19** The winking owl sign of pedicle loss due to spinal metastasis. On an AP radiograph of the lumbar spine, the pedicles should align with those above and below. The vertebral body resembles an owl, with pedicles as the eyes and the spinous process as the beak. A winking owl with an absent pedicle ① is sign of bony destruction.

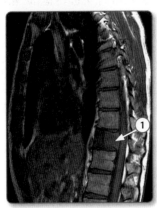

**Figure 3.20** Sagittal MRI scan showing signal change in the T10 vertebral body as a consequence of tumour infiltration.

## Management

Management is operative or nonoperative depending on the risks and benefits of surgery, possible gains versus possible side effects, and any complications.

**Conservative management** Management depends on the stage of the cancer and the prognosis. Radiotherapy is used for pain management and if patients are too unwell or otherwise not suitable candidates for surgery. Radiotherapy is often preferred, especially in cases of no nerve involvement or risk of fracture.

**Surgical management** Surgery is used to decompress the spine or stabilise an affected area. The aims are usually to improve function, stabilise the area and relieve pain.

## 3.8 Other conditions

### Neurogenic shock

Neurogenic shock is caused by impairment of the descending sympathetic pathways, and is associated with acute spinal cord injury. It results in loss of sympathetic innervation to the heart and loss of vasomotor tone, with consequent hypotension and bradycardia. Blood pressure may remain low despite the administration of fluids, and overload is possible with aggressive fluid resuscitation. Neurogenic shock is rare in cases of spinal cord injuries below T6.

### Spinal shock

Spinal shock is not shock in the standard sense; rather, it is temporary loss of function below the level of an acute spinal cord injury, with associated hypotension and bradycardia resulting from the loss of sympathetic drive. There is flaccid paralysis and areflexia, as well as an absent bulbocavernosus reflex. The condition usually resolves within 48 h.

# Shoulder

The shoulder is a shallow ball and socket joint with a wide range of movement. This, and its high functionality, leave it vulnerable to injury and degeneration.

## 4.1 Clinical scenario

### Shoulder pain

#### Background

A 26-year-old man fell on his right shoulder when tackled during a rugby game. He immediately complained of right shoulder pain and was unable to move his shoulder. He was taken to the emergency department where he was found to have pain and swelling on palpation, and no movement in his right shoulder, but good movement of the wrists, elbow and hand.

#### History

Apart from this injury, the patient is fit and well. There is no notable past medical history.

#### Examination

On inspection, there is a depression in the area under the deltoid and swelling more distally (see **Figure 4.18**). The patient has virtually no movement at the shoulder joint, but the elbow and wrist are moving well. He is cradling the weight of his injured arm and has reduced sensation over the lateral border of the upper arm.

#### Differential diagnosis

With these examination findings and the mechanism of injury, the following are considered:

- shoulder dislocation or subluxation with or without an associated fracture
- fracture of the humerus
- soft tissue injury, including significant rotator cuff injury

The deformity strongly suggests a dislocation. This may be associated with a fracture. A soft tissue injury, either a full or partial rotator cuff rupture or tear, would also cause deformity, pain and restriction of movement. However, given the acute presentation and mechanism of injury alongside the clinical deformity, a dislocation is the most likely diagnosis.

### Investigations

After a full examination, shoulder radiographs, including axillary views and apical oblique views, are obtained. These show an anterior dislocation. The radiographs show no evidence of a fracture.

In this case a clear dislocation is seen. If no abnormality had been seen a CT scan would have been used to look for fractures not obvious on radiographs and an ultrasound scan used to look for soft tissue injuries.

The axillary nerve runs around the humeral neck (see page 92). Dislocation of the patient's shoulder has caused compression or traction of the nerve, resulting in loss of sensation in the regimental badge distribution (**Figure 4.1**).

The shoulder joint is reduced under light sedation, and further radiographs are obtained to ensure an adequate position. A full neurological examination finds that axillary nerve function is now normal. Accurate documentation of suspected nerve damage is vital, both before and after reduction, to record any changes and at what time damage occured.

Long-term management is use of a broad arm sling for 2–4 weeks, followed by a course of physiotherapy. If the patient

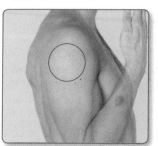

**Figure 4.1** Sensory distribution of the axillary nerve at the shoulder.

has recurrent dislocations, surgical management is considered; early referral to a shoulder specialist is warranted.

## 4.2 Anatomy

The shoulder is a shallow synovial ball-and-socket joint that allows a wide range of movement. Its mobility makes it more unstable than other, more congruent joints, such as the knee or hip.

### Bones

The shoulder consists of the the humerus, scapula and clavicle.

### Humerus

The humerus is the longest bone in the upper limb. It articulates with the scapula at the shoulder, and with the radius and ulnar at the elbow. It has close anatomical relationships with the radial and ulnar nerves, therefore fractures of the humerus often have associated nerve injuries.

In anteroposterior radiographs, the humeral head is not round and symmetrical; it resembles the head of a walking stick. The articular surface of the humerus and the glenoid should be parallel to each other, and the inferior cortices of the acromion and the clavicle should be aligned (**Figures 4.2** and **4.3**).

### Scapula

The scapula is a large, flat, triangular bone that connects the humerus to the clavicle. The glenohumeral joint is at the lateral angle of the scapula, where the glenoid fossa articulates with the head of the humerus (**Figure 4.4**). It is a sturdy bone with a large amount of surrounding muscle, making it generally well protected.

### Clavicle

The clavicle is an 'S'-shaped bone that is widest at the medial end. It acts as a strut bridging the thorax and shoulder. The medial half protects the axillary and subclavian vasculature and the brachial plexus.

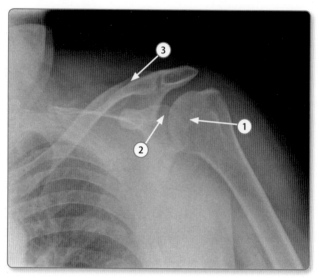

**Figure 4.2** Anteroposterior radiograph of the shoulder, showing relations of the humeral head ①, the glenoid ② and the clavicle ③.

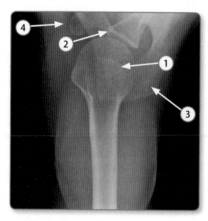

**Figure 4.3** Axial view of the shoulder. The humeral head ① sits on the glenoid ②. The acromion ③ is visible, as is the coracoid process ④.

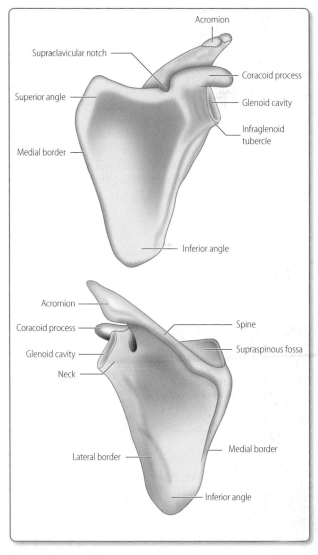

**Figure 4.4** Anatomy of the scapula.

## Articulations

The shoulder has three articulations:

- Glenohumeral joint
- Acromioclavicular joint
- Sternoclavicular joint.

The 'shoulder joint' usually refers to the articulation of the proximal humerus on the glenoid fossa at the glenohumeral joint (**Figure 4.2**).

The glenoid labrum increases the contact area of the glenohumeral joint. Ligamentous structures and the joint capsule further augment static stability. Dynamic stability is provided by local muscles, including the four rotator cuff muscles and the long head of biceps, and extracapsular ligaments.

### The acromioclavicular joint

This is a small synovial joint consisting of the acromion and the distal clavicle. It has minimal mobility, and the surrounding ligaments are integral to the stability of the joint. The acromioclavicular ligament provides horizontal stability, and the coracoclavicular ligament offers vertical stability. The acromioclavicular ligament has superior, inferior, anterior and posterior components, and the coracoclavicular ligament is made up of the trapezoid and conoid ligaments (**Figure 4.5**).

### Clinical insight

In axial view radiographs, the glenoid resembles a golf tee, on top of which the humerus sits like a golfball (**Figure 4.3**). The acromion and coracoid processes look like fingers pointing inferiorly and anteriorly, respectively.

### Rotator cuff

The rotator cuff is a group of muscles that maintain shoulder stability:

- Supraspinatus
- Infraspinatus
- Teres minor
- Subscapularis

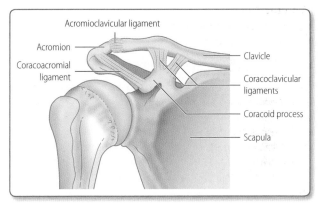

**Figure 4.5** Anatomy of the acromioclavicular joint.

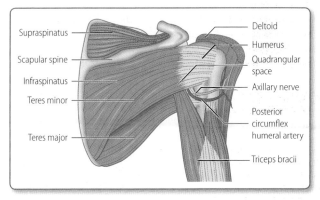

**Figure 4.6** The rotator cuff.

They also initiate abduction, and internal and external rotation of the shoulder. The tendinous parts form the cuff itself (**Figure 4.6**).

## Vascular supply and innervation

Vascular supply of the shoulder and supporting muscles is mainly from the anastomotic ring arising from the anterior and

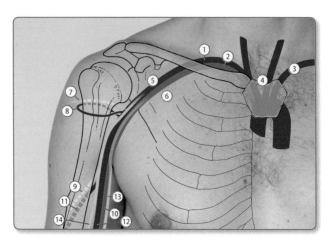

**Figure 4.7** Main neurovasculature of the axilla and arm. (1) Right subclavian artery, (2) right subclavian vein, (3) left subclavian artery, (4) brachiocephalic trunk, (5) axillary artery and approximate position of brachial plexus, (6) axillary vein, (7) axillary nerve, (8) circumflex humeral arteries, (9) radial nerve, (10) brachial vein, (11) profunda brachii artery, (12) brachial artery, (13) ulnar nerve, (14) median nerve.

posterior circumflex humeral arteries, which themselves arise from the axillary artery (**Figure 4.7, Figure 4.24**).

The shoulder joint is closely related posteriorly to the brachial plexus (root values C5–T1). Five nerves originate in the plexus: musculocutaneous, median, ulnar, axillary and radial. The axillary nerve winds round the neck of the humerus and is prone to injury in shoulder dislocations.

### Brachial plexus

The brachial plexus is a network of nerve fibres from nerve roots C5–T1 that innervate the upper limb and pectoral girdle (**Figure 4.8**). It passes through the neck posterior to the subclavian artery, then winds around the axillary artery to enter the limb. Its main branches arise in the axilla. Knowledge of the motor and sensory function of each nerve

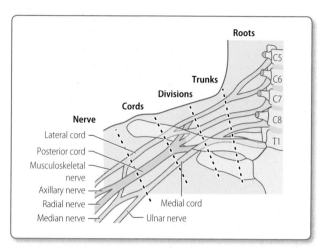

**Figure 4.8** The brachial plexus

| Injury | Nerve affected | Nerve function |
|---|---|---|
| Shoulder dislocation | Axillary nerve | Sensation over regimental badge area |
| Mid-shaft humeral fracture | Radial nerve | Wrist and forearm extension and reduced sensation in the 1st web space |
| Distal humeral fracture | Ulnar nerve | Sensation and flexion of little finger and lateral half of ring finger; interosseous muscles of the hand (fine movements) |

**Table 4.1** Upper limb injuries and associated nerve damage.

is helpful when assessing for neurological deficit after injury (**Table 4.1**).

## Surface anatomy
Many of the bones associated with the shoulder can be palpated easily on examination (**Figures 4.9, 4.10** and **4.11**).

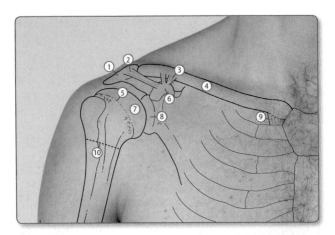

**Figure 4.9** Shoulder joint and anterior pectoral girdle ligaments. ① Acromion, ② coracoacromial ligament, ③ coracoclavicular ligament, ④ clavicle, ⑤ anatomical neck of humerus, ⑥ coracoid process, ⑦ humeral head, ⑧ glenoid fossa, ⑨ costoclavicular ligament, ⑩ surgical neck of humerus.

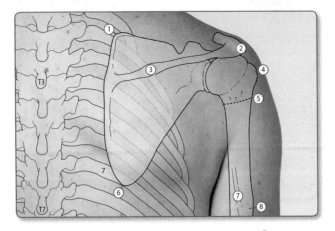

**Figures 4.10** Posterior view of pectoral girdle, shoulder and arm. ① Superior angle, ② angle of the acromion, ③ deltoid tubercle of scapula spine, ④ greater tuberosity, ⑤ surgical neck of humerus, ⑥ inferior angle, ⑦ spiral groove of humerus, ⑧ deltoid tuberosity.

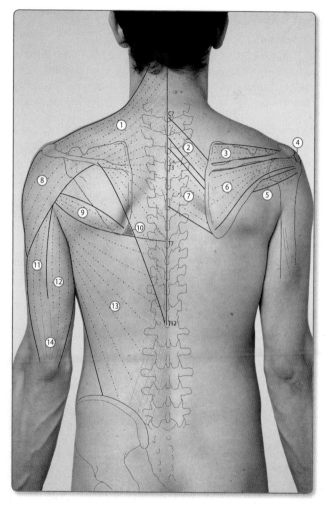

**Figures 4.11** Muscles of the scapula, shoulder and rotator cuff. ① Trapezius, ② rhomboid minor, ③ supraspinatus, ④ supraspinatus tendon, ⑤ teres minor, ⑥ infraspinatus, ⑦ rhomboid major, ⑧ deltoid, ⑨ teres major, ⑩ triangle of auscultation (orange), ⑪ triceps lateral head, ⑫ triceps long head, ⑬ latissimus dorsi, ⑭ triceps tendon.

## 4.3 Examination

### Key signs

Key signs to assess for include muscle wasting, arm posture, asymmetry, reduced range of movement, tenderness, neurological abnormalities, rotator cuff pathology and instability (**Table 4.2**).

### Examination sequence

Examination follows a system of 'look, feel and move', as well as assessment of function, starting proximally and moving distally.

| Test | Tests for | Description |
|------|-----------|-------------|
| Painful arc | Impingement or supraspinatus tendonitis | Positive if pain during active abduction from 60–120° |
| Gerber lift off test | Subscapularis | Dorsum of hand placed over small of the back. Mild resistance applied: if patient is unable to 'lift off' the test is positive |
| Scarf test | Acromioclavicular joint compression | Ipsilateral hand placed on contralateral shoulder, mild pressure pushes arm in. Test positive if pain in acromioclavicular joint |
| Speed's test | Bicep tendonitis | Elbow extended, arm supinated and flexed to 45°. Patient resists downward pressure. Test positive if pain in biceps |
| Neer's sign | Impingement | Positive if pain on passive abduction of shoulder with arm in plane of scapula and internally rotated |
| Hawkins–Kennedy test | Subacromial impingement | Arm held at 90° and the elbow flexed to 90°, arm steadied. Positive if pain on internal rotation |
| Jobe relocation test | Anterior instability | Arm abducted and externally rotated until patient experiences apprehension or discomfort. Test repeated with posterior force applied to humeral head. If range of motion greater in latter, test is positive for anterior instability |

**Table 4.2** Common tests to perform during a shoulder examination.

## Look

- Assess shape, symmetry and colour; look for bruising, swelling and erythema
- Is there any deformity of the joint or tenting of the skin
- Is there any muscle wasting?
- What is the posture of the rest of the arm, elbow and hand?

## Feel

- Palpate for bony tenderness, including along the clavicle, acromioclavicular joint, sternoclavicular joint and all borders of the scapula
- Palpate the greater tuberosity of the humerus
- Palpate the joint space, both anteriorly and posteriorly
- Palpate the muscle for bulk, tenderness, tone and wasting

## Move

- Look for a full range of movement in flexion, extension, adduction, abduction and internal and external rotation (**Figure 4.12**)
- Test movements actively, passively and restricted against your own force to gauge the patient's ability and power

## Function

- What is the patient's range of movement? Can they reach a high shelf or brush their hair? Can they reach up behind their back?

## 4.4 Clavicular fractures

These fractures are classified based on the part of the clavicle they involve:

- Group I clavicular fractures (80% of cases) involve the middle third
- Group II clavicular fractures (15% of cases) involve the lateral third
- Group III clavicular fractures (5% of cases) involve the medial third

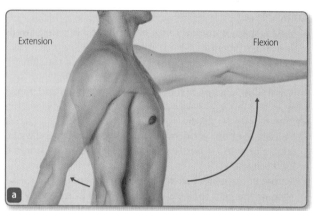

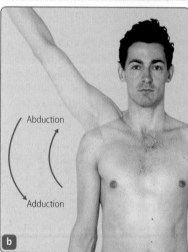

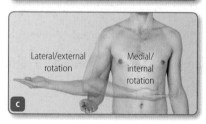

**Figure 4.12** Shoulder movements. (a) Extension/flexion (no ranges), (b) abduction (180–195°), (c) external rotation (45–60°), internal rotation (>90°).

## Epidemiology

Clavicular fractures account for 5–10% of all fractures and up to two thirds of all shoulder fractures. They are most common in the young, active population.

## Causes

Almost 90% of clavicular fractures are caused by a fall on to a shoulder. The other 10% are caused by a direct impact or fall on to an outstretched hand.

## Clinical features

Clinical features include pain, swelling and a reduced range of movement. Redness, bruising and tenting may be seen. Tenting of the skin is caused by upward displacement of the medial portion as a result of the pull of the sternocleidomastoid muscle (**Figure 4.13**).

A neurological examination must be carried out to exclude injury to the brachial plexus, particularly in fractures caused by high-energy trauma. The chest is examined to rule out pneumothorax resulting from apical lung injury.

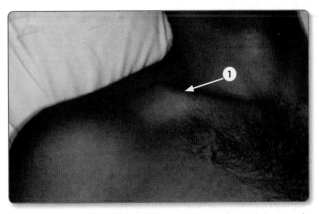

**Figure 4.13** Tenting of the skin caused by prominence and upward elevation of the medial fracture fragment ①.

## Investigations

An anteroposterior radiograph is usually sufficient for diagnosis (**Figure 4.14**). A chest radiograph is obtained if comparison with the contralateral side is needed, and an apical oblique view if displacement is minimal.

Computerised tomography can also be helpful to determine the degree of displacement and comminution, if this is not clear from the radiograph. However, CT is not indicated if it has been decided to manage the fracture conservatively.

## Management

Management depends on the severity and classification of the fracture, and whether it is open or closed.

**Conservative management** Undisplaced, stable fractures with minimal ligamentous injury are managed non-operatively, with use of a broad arm sling and gentle mobilisation starting 2–4 weeks after the injury. A repeat radiograph is done after 6 weeks to check for evidence of healing.

**Surgical management** The following are indications for surgical management:

- Open fracture

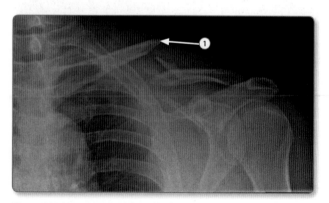

**Figure 4.14** Anteroposterior radiograph of the shoulder showing a high-energy mid-shaft clavicular fracture ①.

- Skin tenting
- Neurovascular injury
- > 100% displacement
- > 2 cm of shortening
- Painful non-union after conservative treatment
- Multiple rib fractures in cases of polytrauma (to help with pain management)

Surgery consists of open reduction and internal fixation with plate and screws, intramedullary nails or a hook plate (**Figure 4.15**).

**Complications** The risks of complications depend on the severity and management of the fracture. The greater the degree of displacement, the higher the risk of malunion or non-union. With open fractures, the risk of infection is much higher. About 9% of clavicular fractures are associated with other fractures, and pneumothorax is present in 3%. Group II fractures are associated with higher rates of non-union.

Complications include:
- Neurovascular injury, caused by the injury or perioperatively

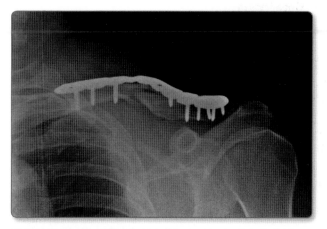

**Figure 4.15** Anteroposterior radiograph of the shoulder showing plate fixation of a mid-shaft fracture of the left clavicle.

- Non-union
- Post-traumatic arthritis
- Pain, irritation and neurovascular injury caused by metal-work in cases managed surgically

# 4.5 Acromioclavicular joint injuries

Acromioclavicular joint injuries commonly occur in active young adults, who suffer injures such as falling from a bicycle. Strong ligaments stabilise the joint (**Figure 4.5**). Depending on the force applied varying degrees of damage to the ligaments occur, from sprains to dissociations of the joint.

## Epidemiology

Acromioclavicular joint injuries are most common in men in their twenties. They make up 9% of all shoulder injuries.

## Causes

These injuries are most commonly caused by direct trauma, for example a fall on to a shoulder. A fall on to an outstretched hand can also cause this injury, but is less common.

## Clinical features

To ensure that any deformity or asymmetry can be seen, the patient is examined while sitting or standing. On palpation, bony tenderness and a 'step off' are felt at the acromioclavicular joint. Tenting of the skin may also be present, and pain limits the range of movement.

## Investigations

Bilateral anteroposterior radiographs are used for direct comparison with the contralateral side to exclude any incidental anatomical findings. An axillary radiograph is used to identify posterior displacement (**Figure 4.16**).

## Management

Management of acromioclavicular joint injuries depends on their severity, whether it is is open or closed and the integrity of the ligaments.

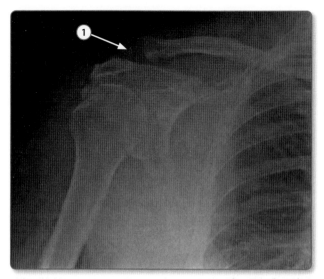

**Figure 4.16** Anteroposterior radiograph showing dislocation of the acromioclavicular joint of the right shoulder. Note the widening of the joint ①, consistent with the injury.

**Conservative management**  For stable, closed injuries, non-operative management consists of rest and 3 weeks in a sling. The aim is for motion by 6 weeks and a return to full mobility by 12 weeks.

**Surgical management**  Surgical management is with open reduction and internal fixation, with or without ligament repair. Surgery is indicated if there is a large amount of displacement; it is also considered if the displacement is moderate but the patient is very active.

**Complications**  Acromioclavicular joint arthritis, distal clavicular osteolysis and chronic subluxation are all complications that follow fractures of the acromioclavicular joint. Any long-term complications are usually tolerated well. However, if pain and reduced function are significant, surgical fixation is considered.

## 4.6 Scapular fractures

The scapula is well protected by surrounding muscles, making fractures rare. Generally scapula fractures are caused by high-energy trauma and part of a pattern of injury that includes the lung and ribs. Scapula fractures are split into those involving the glenoid or those confined to the body; body fractures require no specific treatment.

### Epidemiology

Scapular fractures are uncommon, making up < 1% of all fractures. High-energy injuries have a mortality rate of 2–5%.

### Causes

Significant energy is needed to cause a scapular fracture. Therefore they are usually the result of road traffic accidents or direct trauma from a fall or blunt force.

### Clinical features

The typical clinical features of a scapula fracture are:
- Pain
- Tenderness
- Swelling
- Reduced range of movement

### Investigations

There should be a high index of suspicion, because 80–90% of scapular fractures are associated with other injuries:
- Rib fractures (50% of cases)
- Clavicular fractures (25% or cases)
- Pulmonary contusions (40% of cases)
- Pneumothorax (30% of cases)

Therefore a full, thorough secondary survey is required.

A chest radiograph as part of the trauma series may be the first radiological evidence of a scapular fracture. If a scapular fracture is suspected, an axillary view radiograph and scapula (Y view) are also obtained (**Figure 4.17**). If there is an intra-articular fracture or significant displacement, CT is indicated.

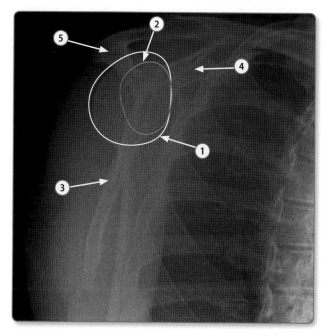

**Figure 4.17** Normal scapula (Y view) showing the humeral head ① sitting over the glenoid ②. The 'Y' is formed by the body ③, coracoid ④ acromion ⑤ of the scapula.

## Management

Most scapular fractures are treated conservatively. Non-operative management consists of use of a sling to support the arm for 2 weeks, analgesia and early gentle mobilisation. Most fractures heal within 6 weeks.

Indications for surgery (open reduction and internal fixation) are:
- Glenohumeral instability
- Displaced scapular neck
- Open fracture
- Loss of rotator function

**Complications**  Associated injuries are usually a greater cause for concern and result in the most serious complications. Malunion can occur with conservative management, but it is generally well tolerated.

## 4.7 Shoulder dislocations

The shoulder is the joint most commonly dislocated, and dislocation is one of the commonest shoulder injuries.

### Epidemiology

Shoulder dislocations are most common in young men (aged 18–30 years) and older women (aged 60–80 years). Younger patients have the highest recurrence rates.

Anterior dislocations are much more common (> 90%) than posterior dislocations. Inferior dislocation (luxatio erecta) may also occur; however, this type of injury is very rare (< 5% of all shoulder dislocations).

### Causes

Anterior dislocations are usually traumatic, caused by:
- direct trauma, i.e. direct impact from behind;
- indirect trauma, i.e. abduction and external rotation, usually after a fall.

Seizures or electric shocks commonly cause posterior dislocations. Recurrent instability may be a consequence of congenital hyperlaxity. If this is the case, very little force is required to cause dislocation and dislocations may be recurrent. Repeated shoulder dislocations as a consequence of trauma give rise to instability.

### Clinical features

The mechanism of injury should be ascertained, as well as whether the dislocation is acute or chronic, and whether it is a first presentation or recurrent. This information guides the investigations and management.

The patient typically presents with severe pain and is unable to move their arm. In anterior dislocations, the arm is usually

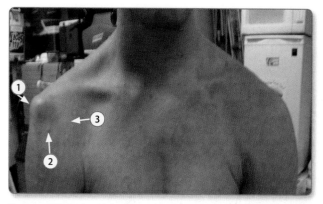

**Figure 4.18** Right shoulder dislocation. There is squaring-off with loss of the normal deltoid contour ① and a sulcus ② caused by the humeral head ③ dislocating anteriorly and medially.

in an abducted position; the shoulder looks square, and a sulcus is seen (**Figure 4.18**). In posterior dislocations, the arm is held in internal rotation and the humeral head is palpable posteriorly.

> ## Clinical insight
>
> The apprehension test is performed by passively abducting, extending and externally rotating the shoulder. The result is positive if the patient complains of pain and says it feels like the shoulder will dislocate.

A full upper limb neurovascular examination is indicated; sensation over the deltoid area may be deficient due to axillary nerve damage (**Figure 4.1**). If the patient is not in acute pain, the dislocation may have spontaneously reduced; an apprehension test should be performed.

### Investigations

Anteroposterior and axillary or Y views are obtained (**Figures 4.2** and **4.3**). Both views must be scrutinised.

**Anterior dislocations**  In anterior dislocations:

- the head of the humerus lies under the coracoid process on the anteroposterior view (**Figure 4.19**);
- the axial view shows the humerus anterior to the glenoid;

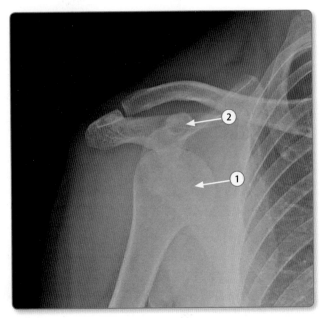

**Figure 4.19** Anteroposterior radiograph showing anterior dislocation of the right shoulder. The joint is no longer congruent. The head of the humerus ① lies under the coracoid process ②.

- the Y view shows the head of the humerus displaced anteriorly so that it no longer covers the glenoid (the centre of the 'Y').

Associated fractures are looked for, including fracture of the greater tuberosity, glenoid fracture (bony Bankart lesion), compression fracture of the posterolateral aspect of the humeral head (Hill–Sachs lesion) and fracture of the acromion or coracoid. The presence of

## Guiding principle

In Y view radiographs, the humeral head should overlie the centre of the glenoid (**Figure 4.14**). The 'Y' is formed by the junction of the body, coracoid and acromion of the scapula.

The junction formed by the stem and the limbs of the 'Y' indicates the centre of the glenoid. The centre of the humerus should overlap this junction.

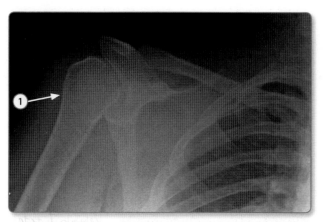

**Figure 4.20** Anteroposterior radiograph showing posterior dislocation of the right shoulder. The humeral head ① appears globular; this is the so-called light bulb sign.

associated fractures alters management and is an indication for surgery.

**Posterior dislocations** In posterior dislocations:
- the head of the humerus appears symmetrical or rounded (the light bulb sign) on the anteroposterior view (**Figure 4.20**);
- the axial view shows the humerus posterior to the glenoid;
- the Y view shows the head of the humerus displaced posteriorly to the junction of the 'Y' (**Figure 4.21**).

## Management
Shoulder dislocations need to be reduced urgently. This is done immediately with analgesia and light sedation, if necessary. If it is a complex and/or irreducible dislocation, the patient requires a manipulation under anaesthesia. After reduction the patient is either treated non-operatively or with an elective procedure, depending on any associated injuries to the shoulder.

**Conservative management** Dislocations are urgently reduced in the emergency department, with the provision of

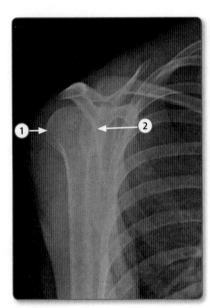

**Figure 4.21** Y view showing a posteriorly dislocated shoulder. The humeral head ① sits posterior to the glenoid ②.

Resusitate
Reduce
Open
Closed
Immobilie
sling
Rehabilitate

analgesia, sedation and in-line traction. Various methods have been described including: the Kocher, Hippocratic and Stimson methods. In general, gentle, prolonged in-line traction will effect reduction. The neurovascular status of the limb, and particularly the axillary nerve, must be documented before reduction.

If an associated fracture is present, administration of general anaesthesia and reduction in an operating theatre with an image intensier is often a better option. This is because it may not be possible to reduce the dislocation in the emergency department; the patient may not be sufficiently relaxed, and rarely soft tissue is interposed in the joint.

After reduction, a repeat anteroposterior radiograph is obtained to confirm reduction. The patient is placed in a broad arm or 'polysling', and their neurological status documented again.

If the dislocation is a patient's first, conservative management usually suffices. Patients are referred to an upper limb surgeon, regardless of the initial management regimen. Patients remain immobilised for 2–4 weeks. Physiotherapy is then started to restore the normal range of shoulder movement.

If a patient has recurrent dislocations and is unable to benefit from extensive immobilisation after reduction, referral to an upper limb surgeon is appropriate to discuss surgical options.

**Surgical management**   If the shoulder cannot be reduced in theatre using a closed approach, or if there is a displaced fracture of the greater tuberosity or glenoid, an open procedure is urgently required. Patients are immobilised postoperatively for 2–3 weeks using a sling and body strap in order to minimise movement. They are then advised to gradually start moving the shoulder out of the sling to improve their strength and range of motion.

Recurrent dislocations require surgery to stabilise the shoulder. This is usually done electively, and further imaging may first be required.

**Complications**   Complications of shoulder dislocations include:
- Recurrence
- Subluxation
- Associated fractures
- Soft tissue injuries, for example rotator cuff tears
- Nerve injury, for example musculocutaneous and axillary nerve injury

## 4.8 Rotator cuff injuries

The tendons of the rotator cuff muscles (**Figure 4.22**) are prone to injury. They can be torn or impinged, leading to pain and restricted movement of the arm. They have varying degrees of severity: some cause only mild reductions in movement that patients can compensate for, while others cause severe pain and loss of function.

### Epidemiology

Rotator cuff injuries are most common in the elderly. However, they are increasingly common in younger, athletic patients.

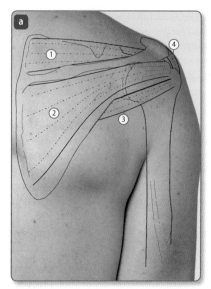

**Figure 4.22** The rotator cuff. (a) Muscles: ① supraspinatus, ② infraspinatus, ③ teres minor, ④ supraspinatus tendon. (b) Tendious insertions of the rotator cuff to the humeral head.

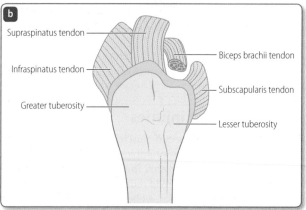

## Causes

In the elderly, rotator cuff impingement and tears are the result of chronic degeneration, most commonly to the supraspinatus tendon under the acromion. In the younger population, these injuries are secondary to repetitive overuse. They are common in people practising activities requiring throwing, explosive or weight-bearing actions, for example baseball pitchers, weightlifters, rugby players and kayakers. Acute subscapularis injuries also occur in younger patients as a consequence of a fall.

### Clinical features

Patients typically present with shoulder pain exacerbated by overhead activities and night pain. On examination, they have reduced abduction and weakness in external rotation and internal rotation, depending on which muscle is affected.

### Investigations

Radiographs occasionally show calcification of the tendons. In severe rotator cuff arthropathy, radiographs show glenohumeral joint degeneration. US has a use in confirming a diagnosis of rotator cuff tears and whether just one tendon or a combination of tendons are involved. MRIs with or without arthrography is useful for a detailed view of the joint and all soft tissues.

### Management

**Conservative management** Rotator cuff injuries are initially managed with activity modification, analgesia, corticosteroid injections and physiotherapy to improve the strength of the muscles.

**Surgical management** Surgery is performed in younger patients whose non-operative management has failed. Repair or reconstruction is unlikely to succeed in older patients because of the level of degeneration, although arthroplasty can be considered. The surgical approach used depends on the pathology, and includes subacromial decompression and or rotator cuff repair. These procedures are usually carried out arthroscopically rather than as open procedures.

For chronic rotator cuff arthropathy, the main problem is migration of the humeral head proximally along with established shoulder arthritis. Arthroplasty of the shoulder is often the preferred treatment, on the basis that the cuff tissue has degenerated to the extent that any attempt to repair it will fail.

**Complications**  Complications of rotator cuff injuries include:
- Recurrence
- Chronic symptoms, including pain
- Reduced range of movement
- Injuries of the axillary and suprascapular nerves

# 4.9 Proximal humeral fractures

Proximal humerus fractures are relatively common injuries, usually caused by low-impact falls in the elderly or high-energy trauma in the young.

## Epidemiology
Proximal humeral fractures are the most common humeral fractures in adults. Their incidence is increased incidence in elderly women.

## Causes
This type of injury is commonly caused by a fall from standing height on to an outstretched arm in elderly patients with osteoporosis. In young patients, it is more likely to be caused by high-energy trauma, for example in a road traffic accident.

The proximal humerus is a common site of bony metastases, so it can be a site of pathological fractures. Seizures and electric shocks are rare causes of proximal humeral fracture.

## Clinical features
Patients present with shoulder or arm pain. The shoulder and upper arm, and even the chest wall, are usually swollen and bruised. Bony tenderness is present, and the range of motion is severely reduced because of pain.

Upper limb neurological function is assessed, especially sensation in the distribution of the axillary nerve.

## Investigations
Standard shoulder radiographs are obtained, including anteroposterior, lateral and axillary views. CT scans, especially

with three-dimensional reconstruction views, are useful if the fracture is comminuted and in more than two parts.

## Management

There are many different fracture patterns of proximal humeral fractures, classified according to the number of parts affected: the humeral neck, humeral shaft, greater tuberosity and lesser tuberosity (**Figure 4.23**). These four parts are the foundation of the Neer classification (types I–VI); however, in this classification a part is defined as displaced only if there is > 1 cm displacement or > 45° angulation.

The Neer classification enables prognostication regarding the outcome of treatment, e.g. four-part fractures have a poor prognosis and a high chance of developing osteonecrosis.

Knowledge of the neurovascular anatomy of the humerus is essential, because damage to vessels, including the arcuate artery (**Figure 4.24**), can lead to avascular necrosis.

A full history from the patient is necessary, because management decisions are based on it. Specfically ask:
- What is the patient's normal level of activity?

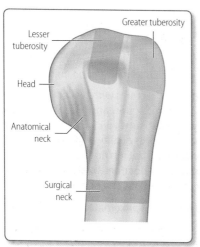

Figure 4.23 Anatomy of the proximal humerus.

Greater tuberosity

Lesser tuberosity

Head

Anatomical neck

Surgical neck

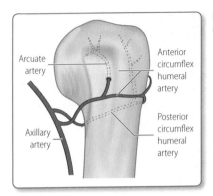

**Figure 4.24** Neurovascular anatomy of the humerus.

- Which is their dominant hand?
- Do they have any other injuries?
- How are they likely to respond to any rehabilitation regimen?

**Conservative management** For most one-part fractures, conservative management with collar-and-cuff immobilisation is adequate. Regular reviews are needed to check the position of the fracture. Early mobilisation with pendulum exercises is recommended as early as 2 weeks after the injury. After 6 weeks, patients start a full range of active movements.

In elderly patients, severely displaced or angulated fractures may be treated conservatively, and a good result is usually achieved. However, they are warned that some restrictions of their range of motion, particularly abduction, may remain.

**Surgical management** Most fractures with two or more parts (**Figure 4.25**) require open reduction and internal fixation (**Figure 4.26**), especially if the patient is young, because improving function significantly improves quality of life. Hemiarthroplasty (**Figure 4.27**) can be used, but it is normally a secondary option after failure of open reduction. In elderly patients, hemiarthroplasty may be carried out as a primary procedure.

**Complications** Complications of proximal humeral fractures include:
- Avascular necrosis

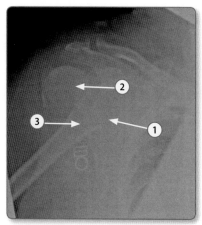

**Figure 4.25** Anterioposterior radiograph showing displaced fracture of the proximal humerus ①. The humeral head ② is in the joint. The fracture is clearly visible because of the significant displacement of the humerus ③ distal to the fracture.

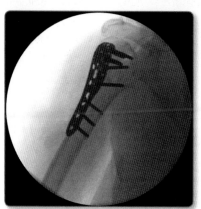

**Figure 4.26** Intraoperative radiograph showing plating of a proximal humeral fracture.

- Stiffness
- Osteoarthritis
- Injuries of the axillary artery and brachial plexus
- Non-union
- Malunion
- Injuries of the axillary and suprascapular nerves

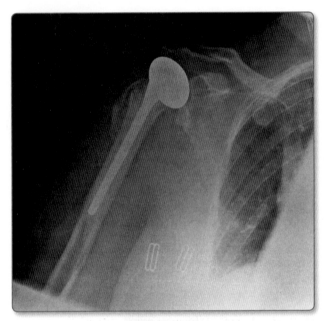

**Figure 4.27** Shoulder hemiarthroplasty carried out as primary fracture management in an elderly patient with a comminuted proximal humeral fracture.

## 4.10 Humeral shaft fractures

Humeral shaft fractures occur in the diaphysis of the humerus. They are associated with neurapraxia and are inherently unstable, usually requiring fixation.

### Epidemiology

Humeral shaft fractures account for around 3% of all fractures. They occur most commonly in young men as a result of trauma and elderly women from low-velocity falls.

### Causes

The most common mechanism of injury is direct trauma from a blow or road traffic accident, which leads to transverse or comminuted fractures. Spiral or oblique fractures are more likely in elderly patients, and occur as a result of falls or twisting injuries.

### Clinical features

Fractures of the humeral shaft typically present with pain, swelling, deformity, weakness and shortening of the arm. The fracture may be an open injury if secondary to trauma or part of polytrauma.

The neurovascular structures are examined. Assessment of radial nerve function is required; damage is indicated by wrist drop and loss of sensation on the dorsum of the hand.

### Investigations

Anteroposterior and lateral radiographs of the humerus are obtained (**Figure 4.28**), as well as radiographs of the shoulder and elbow joints to rule out intra-articular extension. CT, bone scans and MRI are required if the fracture is particularly

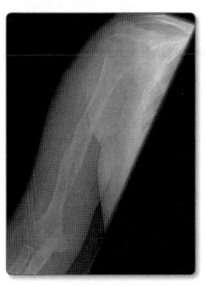

**Figure 4.28**
Anteroposterior radiograph of a humerus showing a right-sided spiral mid-shaft humeral fracture in a young man.

comminuted or if soft tissues need to be viewed in more detail. The fracture is described according to:

- whether it is open or closed;
- location (proximal, middle or distal third);
- whether it is displaced or non-displaced;
- fracture pattern.

## Management

The aim of treatment is bony union with good alignment. Acceptable alignment is:

- < 20° anterior angulation
- < 30° varus or valgus angulation
- < 3 cm of shortening

As with most fractures, both fracture characteristics and the circumstances of the patient need to be taken into account when deciding between management options.

**Conservative management** Most humeral shaft fractures (> 90%) are treated conservatively with close monitoring and follow-up in the fracture clinic. The humerus tolerates deformity much better than most other bones, because of the degree of movement afforded by the shoulder.

Different immobilisation methods are available, including use of a hanging cast or U-slab. This is replaced with a humeral brace 1–2 weeks after the injury. The brace must be compressed every 1–2 weeks to maintain the stiffness of the fractured segment and bring the fragments closer together. Braces maintain fracture alignment but allow movement of the shoulder and elbow joints, thereby preventing stiffness. Braces are usually worn for 6–8 weeks, until radiographs confirm union.

**Surgical management** Indications for open reduction and internal fixation are:

- Failed closed management (e.g. non-union or malunion)
- Polytrauma
- Open fractures
- Pathological fractures
- Segmental fractures

- Fractures with associated nerve or vascular injury
- Fractures with an intra-articular component

Optimum management, with the best functional outcome, is with open reduction and plate fixation. Intramedullary nails are used for pathological fractures, fractures in osteoporotic bone and extensive segmental fractures. However, intramedullary nailing is associated with shoulder pain, nerve injuries and non-union. If the fracture is open and there is extensive soft tissue injury, external fixation is another option.

**Complications** Common complications of humeral shaft fractures are:

- Injury to the radial nerve
- Malunion
- Non-union

## 4.11 Brachial plexus injuries

The brachial plexus (**Figure 4.8**) is susceptible to injury because of its long course. Injuries and lesions can lead to severe functional impairment.

### Epidemiology

Newborns (5 in every 1000 births) and young men are commonly affected by brachial plexus injuries. Around 1% of polytrauma patients have a brachial plexus injury.

### Causes

In children, brachial plexus injuries are caused by traction on the arm during breech delivery or other complicated birth (e.g. cases of shoulder dystocia). In adults, lesions result from violent falls on the side of the head and shoulder, forcing the two apart and putting strain on the upper roots of the plexus. Typical mechanisms of injury are falls from trees, high-speed motorcycle accidents, falls and traction injuries with forced abduction on the arm, and gunshot or stab wounds. Very rarely, lesions are the consequence of brachial neuritis (Parsonage–Turner syndrome).

## Clinical features

The patient complains of pain and sensory loss in the limb. In severe cases, their arm may be hanging flail at their side, and they may have bruising over the shoulder or at the base of the neck.

A thorough neurological examination is necessary to ascertain which myotomes, dermatomes and roots are involved. Is the lesion nerve preganglionic or postganglionic? Does the patient have oculosympathetic palsy (Horner's syndrome, i.e. ptosis, small pupil and absence of sweating on the affected side)? This represents disruption of the sympathetic chain via C8–T1 avulsions, and therefore a preganglionic lesion. Muscles to test are the serratus anterior and rhomboids; if they are functioning, postganglionic injury is most likely.

Associated injuries are always sought, for example injuries of the head, neck, chest, abdomen or blood vessels.

The lesion can be at any level (spinal cord, root, trunk, etc.). Two classic types of palsy result from brachial plexus injury.

- Erb–Duchenne palsy is caused by damage at C5 and C6 (the upper roots of the brachial plexus): the arm hangs at the patient's side, internally rotated, adducted and with a flexed wrist (the so-called waiter's tip)
- Klumpke's palsy is caused by damage at C8 and T1 (the lower roots of the brachial plexus): the hand is clawed, and there may be sympathetic trunk involvement leading to Horner's syndrome

In severe injuries, all roots may be injured.

## Investigations

Radiographs of the cervical spine and chest are obtained. CT or MRI scans assess whether there is nerve root avulsion from the cord (preganglionic injury). Electromyography is used to test motor and sensory activity, and thereby help distinguish preganglionic from postganglionic injuries. The histamine test can be used to test for postganglionic damage.

## Management

Most brachial plexus injuries are managed non-operatively. Nerves regenerate at a rate of 1 mm per day, so improvements can naturally occur over time.

**Conservative management**
This consists of observation and waiting for recovery. If no electromyographic abnormalities are apparent at 3–4 weeks, the prognosis is good with conservative treatment including intensive physiotherapy. However, the patient is warned that recovery can take years.

> ### Guiding principle
>
> In the histamine test, a drop of 1% histamine is placed over the centre of each dermatome and the skin is pricked through it. The normal side is the control and should show a flare. Absence of a flare on the injured side indicates postganglionic nerve injury.

**Surgical management** Open injuries are explored acutely if the patient's condition is stable and they have no other, more life-threatening injuries. Delayed surgery is required for most patients with a traumatic injury; this can be done at 3–6 months after injury, at a specialist nerve injury unit. Recovery generally takes years and is usually unsatisfactory. Recover from some injuries may not be possible, in which case tendon transfers is considered to restore some useful upper limb function.

**Complications** Irreparable motor or sensory deficits are the potential complications of brachial plexus injuries.

## 4.12 Biceps tendon injuries

Biceps tendon injuries present with tendon pain (especially acute pain) at the shoulder and reduction in range of movement.

### Clinical features

Patients present with sudden-onset anterior shoulder pain and a 'pop' after playing sport or using weights in the gym. In the history, steroid use is asked about specifically because there is an association between the two due to the increased strain and state of chronic inflammation.

The patient may have a Popeye deformity. This is caused by the lack of attachment of the long head of the biceps tendon, causing the muscle to bunch and therefore appear as a bulge in the upper arm, much like that of the cartoon character Popeye. Tenderness on palpation in the biceps groove is likely, along with a palpable defect as a consequence of distal migration of the tendon. Pain and loss of strength on flexion of the elbow or supination of the forearm are present.

## Investigations

Ultrasound shows if there is a rupture, whether partial or full thickness, and excludes tendonitis. MRI is the gold standard for imaging.

## Management

In older or more sedentary patients, conservative management in the form of analgesia and physical therapy is the preferred option. However, in younger, more active patients, surgical repair is indicated to prevent any loss of flexion or supination and grip strength.

The elbow is a modified hinge joint, and one of the most stable joints in the body as a result of a high degree of joint congruity (throughout the range of motion of the joint a large amount of contact between the articular surfaces remains) and the support of strong ligaments. The main functions of the elbow are to extend or flex the arm to enable the hand to reach for and manipulate objects, and to transfer energy from the shoulder during activities requiring force, such as throwing.

The elbow may be injured by direct or indirect force. Indirect force is usually a fall onto the hand, whereas direct force implies an injury with impact onto the elbow. Elbow injuries are associated with pain, swelling and reluctance to move the joint. The patient often holds the affected arm into the trunk in an attempt to splint the limb, which results in an abnormal posture. The elbow is frequently deformed with loss of normal contours, particularity if the joint is dislocated. Elbow injuries may be open (when a broken bone breaks through the skin) or closed.

## 5.1 Clinical scenario

### Elbow pain

#### Presentation

A 47-year-old woman presents with pain in her right elbow. She describes it as an aching pain that becomes sharp when she uses the elbow. The pain radiates to the shoulder and into the forearm. Elbow flexion or wrist extension worsens the pain. When it is at its most severe, she occasionally gets a pricking sensation ('pins and needles') in the thumb and index finger. However, she has no other neurological symptoms.

She first noticed the pain about a year ago. She has been prompted to seek help because the pain is becoming more frequent, and during a game of squash last night, it became severe enough to make her stop playing. She recalls no injury.

## History

There is no significant medical history. The patient is a home-maker and enjoys sport, including golf, tennis and squash. She is right-handed.

## Examination

No obvious swelling or deformity is present, but there is mild tenderness over the lateral epicondyle on palpation. There is a good range of movement but general stiffness. The patient has pain on resisted wrist extension and when placing her hand in a grip. Neurological examination is normal.

## Differential diagnosis

Common causes of elbow pain are:
- cervical spine pathology (i.e. nerve impingement)
- radial tunnel syndrome (from nerve entrapment)
- bony injury
- tendon rupture
- osteoarthritis
- inflammatory arthropathy
- lateral epicondylitis (tennis elbow)

The most likely cause of her symptoms is lateral epicondylitis. The history of lateral-sided elbow pain, exacerbated by activity, with the absence of significant neurology would suggest this diagnosis. The examination finding of pain on the resisted wrist extension makes the diagnosis highly likely. The diagnosis of lateral epicondylitis is clinical.

## Investigations

A lateral and anteroposterior radiograph of the elbow are required to exclude bony pathology.

If the results of all imaging studies and blood tests are normal, as in this case, a diagnosis of lateral epicondylitis (tennis elbow) can be made.

The patient is reassured that the condition is self-limiting, and advised to rest the elbow and avoid any activities that exacerbate the pain and associated symptoms for the next 3–6 months. She is offered NSAIDs and an elbow strap, and and will be referred for physiotherapy if the pain continues.

## 5.2 Anatomy

The elbow joint consists of three articulations of the humerus with the radius and ulna (**Figures 5.1** and **5.2**):

- Ulnotrochlear

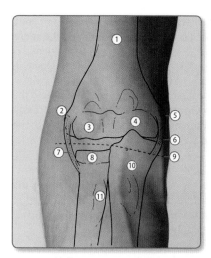

**Figure 5.1** Elbow joint: anterior view. ① Humeral shaft, ② lateral epicondyle, ③ capitulum, ④ trochlea, ⑤ medial epicondyle, ⑥ medial collateral ligament, ⑦ lateral collateral ligament, ⑧ radial head, ⑨ elbow joint line, ⑩ ulna, ⑪ radial tuberosity.

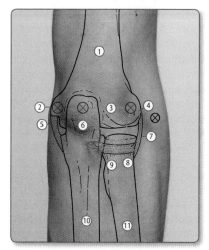

**Figure 5.2** Elbow joint: posterior view. ① Humeral shaft, ② medial epicondyle, ③ borders of anconeus triangle (blue), ④ lateral epicondyle, ⑤ medial collateral ligament, ⑥ olecranon, ⑦ lateral collateral ligament, ⑧ annular ligament surrounding radial head, ⑨ radial neck, ⑩ posterior border of ulna, ⑪ radial shaft, ⊗ horizontal alignment of the epicondyles and olecranon during elbow extension, ⊗ forearm extensor muscle mass.

- Radiocapitellar
- Proximal radioulnar

These are supported by strong ligaments palpable between their attachment points: the lateral (radial) and ulnar (medial) collateral ligaments.

Knowledge of the normal features of elbow bones, and how they are aligned, enables the identification of joint lines, injection sites, nerve positions and the diagnosis of dislocations and fractures.

### Olecranon

The olecranon is the most proximal section of the ulna and the insertion for the triceps. Together with the coronoid process, it makes up a semilunar notch that forms a stable joint with the distal humerus (**Figure 5.2**).

### Vascular supply

The brachial artery passes into the cubital fossa deep to the biceps aponeurosis, before bifurcating at the radial head to form the ulnar and radial arteries. Branches of the brachial artery anastomose to supply the elbow joint.

### Innervation

Branches of many nerves provide the elbow with motor and sensory innervation (**Figure 5.3**). Three nerves have important relationships to the elbow joint:

- The median nerve runs medial to the brachial artery in the cubital fossa, and travels down the forearm to the wrist
- The ulnar nerve passes posterior to the medial epicondyle and continues into the anterior forearm
- The radial nerve passes close to the radiohumeral joint, then divides into superficial and deep (posterior interosseous) branches

## 5.3 Examination

### Key signs

Key signs to assess for include swelling, loss of normal skin contours, deformity in both the coronal and sagittal planes, skin

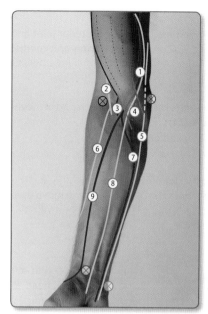

**Figure 5.3**
Neurovasculature of the cubital fossa and forearm. (1) Brachial artery, (2) radial nerve, (3) biceps tendon, (4) biceps aponeurosis, (5) ulnar nerve, (6) superficial branch of radial nerve, (7) ulnar artery, (8) median nerve, (9) radial artery, ⊗ lateral epicondyle, ⊗ medial epicondyle, ⊗ flexor carpi radialis tendon, ⊗ pisiform and flexor carpi ulnaris tendon.

changes, scars, tenderness, fluctuance and restricted range of movement. Look also for abnormalities in the shoulder, wrist and hand on the affected side.

### Examination sequence

Examination follows a system of 'Look, feel and move', and test of function, starting proximally and moving distally.

### Look

- Is there any swelling or bruising?
- Observe the joint from all angles; is there an obvious deformity?
- Are there any open wounds or puncture wounds?
- Scars
- Assess the carrying angle, normally about 7° of valgus for males and 13° for females

## Feel

- Palpate for bony tenderness along the posterior joint line (between the lateral epicondyle, olecranon and medial epicondyle)

## Move

- Assess elbow flexion and extension (normal range of movement, 0–145°) (**Figure 5.4**)
- Assess supination (85°) and pronation (70°)

## Function

- Test the nerves and feel for pulses
- Determine whether or not the patient is able to move their elbow actively

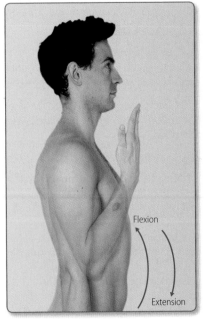

**Figure 5.4** Elbow movements. Flexion (145°) extension (0°).

## 5.4 Elbow dislocation

The elbow may dislocate anteriorly or posteriorly. Most posterior dislocations occur as a consequence of a fall onto an outstretched arm. Elbow dislocations are very painful and may, or may not, be associated with a bony injury. Due to the proximity of nerves and blood vessels around the elbow, neurovascular injury may occur. Look for these injuries and document your findings. Elbow dislocations require prompt reduction.

Elbow dislocations are classed as:

- Simple
- No fracture seen
- Complex (meaning that an associated fracture is present; about 50% of elbow dislocations are classed as complex)

Associated fractures most commonly involve the radial head, with or without the coronoid process of the ulna. Shear fractures of the capitellum are less common. Recurrent dislocations are uncommon.

### Epidemiology

The elbow is the second most common joint to dislocate (the first is the shoulder). Elbow dislocations are most common between the ages of 10 and 20 years, and 80% of dislocations are posterior.

### Causes

Most elbow dislocations are caused by falls on the hand or elbow, or injuries sustained while playing sport. Posterior dislocations occur when the elbow is hyperextended. Anterior dislocations are normally the result of a direct posterior force to a flexed arm.

### Clinical features

The typical clinical features are:

- Deformity
- Swelling and pain
- Reduced range of movement

Nerve injuries are uncommon, but the ulnar and anterior inter-osseous nerves can be damaged because of their proximity to the joint. The brachial artery is also at risk of injury. Therefore a careful neurovascular examination is required before and after reduction of the dislocation and examination of the skin to determine whether the injury is closed or open.

As always, be aware of the risk of compartment syndrome (see page 349).

### Investigations

Anteroposterior and lateral radiographs are required before and after reduction. The dislocation is described in the direction of the displacement of the olecranon relative to the humerus; for example, **Figure 5.5** shows a posterior dislocation. CT may be

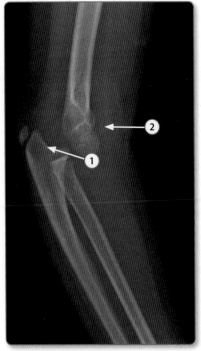

**Figure 5.5** Lateral radiograph showing posterior dislocation of a child's elbow. The olecranon (ulna) ① has displaced posteriorly to the humerus ②.

helpful in assessment of a complex dislocation, and it is needed for preoperative planning.

## Management

The aim is to restore the stability of the elbow. Elbow dislocations associated with one or more intra-articular fractures are at greater risk of recurrent or chronic instability.

**Conservative management** Patients with simple dislocations usually undergo closed reduction under sedation. Reduction is usually achieved by gentle traction and gradual increase in flexion while pushing the olecranon back over the distal humerus. Stability is assessed while the patient remains sedated.

- For a stable simple dislocation, a collar and cuff sling is used for 10 days
- For an unstable simple dislocation, a temporary above-elbow back slab, converted to a hinged elbow brace, is used for 2–3 weeks.

The patient is encouraged to move the elbow as early as able to prevent the joint from becoming stiff.

> ### Clinical insight
>
> The terrible triad fracture must not be missed. It comprises elbow dislocation, radial head fracture and coronoid fracture, and is an extremely unstable injury. Operative fixation of the bony and ligamentous structures may be required to confer stability to the joint. Even then elbow instability may occur. This is why assessment of the radial head and coronoid is essential in any dislocation of the elbow.

**Surgical management** Complex fractures usually require open reduction and internal fixation, with or without repair of the capsule and ligaments. Any open fracture also requires a washout as a minimum and appropriate antibiotics.

**Complications** Elbow dislocations have the following potential complications:

- reduced range of movement, and stiffness
- nerve injury (ulnar nerve and anterior interosseous nerve)
- vascular injury (brachial artery)
- arthritis
- heterotopic ossification (bone formation in an abnormal anatomical site, usually soft tissue)

- compartment syndrome
- instability

## 5.5 Supracondylar fractures (distal humeral fractures)

Distal humeral fractures are a family of fractures that occur at the region of the elbow, and almost always involve the articular surface. The fracture patterns may be vertical or transverse/oblique with varying degrees of comminution. Distal intercondylar fractures are the most common variant. A small proportion of distal humeral fractures are transverse, and are extra-articular. Given that most fractures are intra-articular injuries, the risk of stiffness and post-traumatic arthritis is high.

### Epidemiology

Almost all fractures are caused by direct impact onto the elbow, e.g. a fall. The incidence is bimodal: high energy injuries in young men; and low energy injuries in older women.

### Causes

Supracondylar fractures are often caused by a direct impact to the elbow with high energy. However, in the older population (≥70 years) a low-energy impact may produce a fracture pattern as complex as that caused by a high-energy impact in younger people. The fracture pattern often extends into the articular surface of the distal humerus in a 'Y' or 'T' pattern.

### Clinical features

Distal humerus fractures typically present with:

- pain
- swelling
- bruising
- loss of the normal elbow contour
- reluctance to move the elbow actively or to have it moved passively

## Investigations

Anteroposterior and lateral radiographs of the elbow are necessary. Almost all patients with suspected supracondylar fracture require a CT scan for preoperative planning, because of the complex nature of these injuries (**Figure 5.6**).

## Management

Most supracondylar fractures are managed operatively, because they usually involve articular surfaces.

**Conservative management**  This should be considered when there is little displacement with a fracture that is truly supracondylar, i.e. without extension or displacement into the articular surfaces. As always, patients with significant comorbidities or at increased risk of anaesthesia complications are candidates for non-operative management.

**Surgical management**  Open reduction and internal fixation of the fracture enables accurate reduction of the fracture and restoration of the articular surfaces. The elbow is often

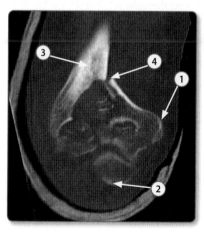

**Figure 5.6** CT scan (coronal view) showing a complex intra-articular intercondylar fracture to the distal humerus. ① Medial epicondyle, ② olecranon, ③ shaft of humerus, ④ complex fracture configuration.

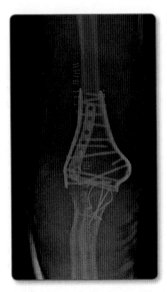

**Figure 5.7** Postoperative radiograph showing plate fixation of a complex distal humerus.

approached via an olecranon osteotomy. The fracture is usually fixed by using two plates, one medial and one lateral. Rigid fixation allows early movement of the elbow joint, thereby helping reduce stiffness. **Figure 5.7** shows plate fixation of a complex supracondylar fracture.

**Complications**  The potential complications of supracondylar fractures are:

- Stiffness
- Nerve injury (ulnar nerve, radial nerve and median nerve)
- Vascular injury
- Non-union
- Heterotopic ossification
- Removal of metalwork
- Osteoarthritis

## 5.6 Olecranon fractures

Olecranon fractures occur usually by direct impact onto the point of the elbow (olecranon) or may occur by indirect force. They are common across all age ranges. The spectrum of injury ranges from an extra-articular avulsion injury to a complex pattern of fracture involving the joint extending into the proximal ulna.

### Epidemiology

Olecranon fractures have a bimodal distribution: they are caused by traumatic, high-energy injuries in a younger age group and falls in the elderly. They usually occur as a result of direct impact.

### Causes

They are caused either as a consequence of a direct impact or an indirect force, often with a powerful contraction of the triceps muscle. Direct impact often results in a comminuted fracture pattern. Indirect force results in a transverse or avulsion pattern.

### Clinical features

Patients with olecranon fractures typically present with:
- pain
- swelling and bruising
- reduced range of movement, especially extension

### Investigations

A full neurovascular examination is essential because of the possibility of damage to the ulnar nerve (see **Figure 5.3**). Anteroposterior and lateral radiographs (**Figures 5.8** and **5.9**, respectively) are required. If the fractured is comminuted, a CT scan is useful to understand the fracture pattern and for preoperative planning.

### Management

With both conservative and surgical management, mobilisation as early as possible is needed to prevent stiffening of the joint.

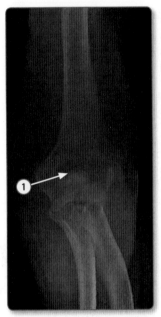

**Figure 5.8** Anteroposterior radiograph of the elbow, showing an olecranon fracture. The olecranon ① is in a more proximal position than would be expected, although the fracture is difficult to discern on this view.

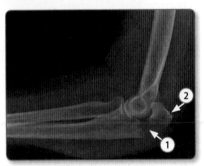

**Figure 5.9** Lateral radiograph of the elbow. The fracture ① is much easier to discern on this view than on the anteroposterior radiograph (Figure 5.8). There is posterior displacement of the olecranon ②.

**Conservative management** Indications for non-operative management are:

- non-displaced fractures
- displaced fractures with low demand, i.e. in older patients with low functional requirement

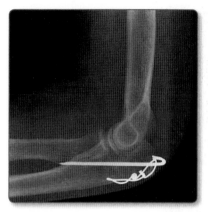

**Figure 5.10** Lateral radiograph of the elbow, showing open reduction and internal fixation of an olecranon fracture, using tension band wiring.

These fractures are treated by immobilisation in a splint, with the elbow held at 90° for 3–4 weeks.

**Surgical management** This consists of open reduction and internal fixation, with either tension band wiring or plates and screws.

> **Clinical insight**
>
> Tension band wiring enables the force produced by the triceps to be converted into a compressive force across the fracture site (**Figure 5.10**).

**Complications** Olecranon fractures have a number of potential complications:

- stiffness (up to 50% of patients)
- non-union
- ulnar nerve injury
- complications caused by metalwork (e.g. pain on resting the elbow because of prominent subcutaneous wires or skin breakdown due to erosion from prominent subcutaneous wires)

## 5.7 Capitellum fractures

Capitellum fractures make up only a small proportion of elbow fractures (1%), and result from a coronal plane fracture of the distal humerus. They present with pain and restricted range of movement. The injury may not be obvious on plain radiographs; CT is required if there is any doubt.

Capitellum fractures are classified as follows.

- Type 1 capitellum fractures are isolated to the capitellum
- Type 2 capitellum fractures have medial extension into the trochlea
- Type 3 capitellum fractures consist of separate capitellum and trochlear fragments

### Causes

This type of fracture occurs when a force is transmitted to the capitellum directly by the radial head with the arm held in a semi-flexed position. The injury is usually the result of a shear force.

### Clinical features

Capitellum fractures typically present with:

- pain
- swelling
- reduced range of motion at the elbow

### Investigations

Anteroposterior (**Figure 5.11**) and lateral radiographs of the elbow are required. A CT scan is usually also needed to fully show the fracture pattern.

### Management

Capitellum fractures are managed surgically unless there is very little displacement or the patient is unfit for surgery.

**Conservative management**  This is used for fractures isolated to the capitellum and with minimal displacement. Treatment consists of above-elbow casting for 6 weeks. The patient initially needs repeat weekly radiographs to ensure that there is no displacement.

**Surgical management**  This is the preferred option for the vast majority of capitellum fractures. It enables accurate restoration of the articular surfaces. Small irreducible fragments are excised. Headless compression screws are used to fix the

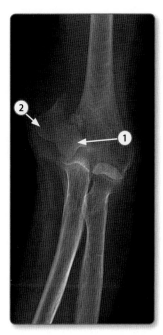

**Figure 5.11** Anteroposterior radiograph of the elbow, showing a type 2 capitellar fracture involving both the capitellum ① and the trochlea ②.

fragments, resulting in minimal irregularity of the articular surface after surgery.

**Complications**  Potential complications include:

- stiffness
- pain
- osteoarthritis
- metalwork problems

## 5.8 Radial head and neck fractures

Radial head and neck fractures are the most common elbow fractures, and are associated with elbow dislocations and/ or ligamentous injury (MCL, LCL). The radial head is a bony constraint to the elbow providing stability to a valgus force.

Even the most undisplaced radial head and neck fractures are associated with a loss of terminal elbow extension.

Mason classified radial head and neck fractures into three types.
- Type 1 fractures have minimal displacement, intra-articular displacement < 2 mm and no block to rotation
- Type 2 fractures have displacement > 2 mm, with or without angulation, and a block to rotation may be present
- Type 3 fractures are displaced, comminuted fractures

### Epidemiology
Radial head and neck fractures occur in 20% of all elbow injuries.

### Causes
The mechanism of injury is usually a fall on to an outstretched hand with transference of force to the radiocapitellar joint.

### Clinical features
Radial head and neck fractures present with:
- pain, especially at the lateral aspect of the elbow
- reduced range of movement of the elbow and forearm

About 30% of radial head fractures have associated injuries: ligament injuries, the terrible triad, coronoid fracture, elbow dislocation or disruption of the distal radioulnar joint. The wrist is palpated to assess the stability of the distal radioulnar joint.

The distal or proximal radioulnar joint may be injured (subluxed or dislocated) with a fracture to the radius or ulna. These specific injury patterns have eponymous nomenclature (**Figure 5.12**).

### Investigations
Anteroposterior (**Figure 5.13**) and lateral radiographs are required, with CT for comminuted fractures.

### Management
As with other fractures involving the elbow joint, mobilisation of the joint as early as possible is a priority to prevent stiffness.

**Conservative management** This approach works well for fractures without displacement or with only minimal displacement.

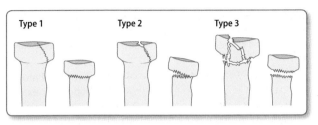

**Figure 5.12** Mason classification of fractures of the radial head and neck.

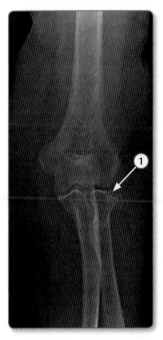

**Figure 5.13** Anteroposterior radiograph of the elbow, showing a type 2 fracture of the radial head ①.

The arm is placed in a sling for 48 h. This is followed by early encouragement of a range of movement as the pain allows.

**Surgical management** This consists of open reduction and internal fixation with or without radial head replacement or excision.

## Guiding principle

There are two specific injury patterns that affect either the proximal or distal radioulnar joint.

- A Monteggia fracture is characterised by radial head dislocation and fracture of the proximal ulna
- A Galeazzi fracture is characterised by disruption of the distal radioulnar joint and fracture of the distal third of the radius

**Complications** The potential complications of radial head and neck fractures are:

- stiffness
- reduced range of movement, especially extension
- instability and pain

Patients are warned that a there may be a block to terminal extension and they may never regain the full straightening at the elbow, even with a non-displaced fracture.

# 5.9 Other conditions

Other conditions of the elbow include soft tissue complaints and more unusual fractures. Soft tissue complaints are common and are usually managed in primary care.

## Coronoid process fractures

The coronoid process is important for anterior stability of the elbow. The coronoid is the bony extension of the anterior ulna and provides an anterior buttress to the elbow joint. It is an intra-articular structure which increases the bony congruency of the elbow joint. The medial collateral ligament attaches onto the ulnar side of the process.

Coronoid process fractures are caused by avulsion of the brachialis origin during hyperextension injuries. They are associated with up to 10% of elbow dislocations and can lead to instability after dislocation.

The three common fracture patterns of the coronoid are:
- simple avulsion
- fractures involving < 50% of the coronoid process
- fractures involving > 50% of the coronoid process

The first two types are treated conservatively with immobilisation for 2–3 weeks. The third type of fracture requires open reduction and internal fixation because of the risk of recurrent dislocation and instability.

## Olecranon bursitis

The olecranon bursa sits on the extensor aspect of the olecranon. It can become inflamed and irritated, resulting in a red, painful swelling over the olecranon. Bursitis can either be infective or non-infective, caused by trauma.

The history guides the choice of investigations, which may include blood tests, radiographs and aspiration. Nearly all cases of olecranon bursitis are treated non-operatively with compression bandage; non-steroidal anti-inflammatory drugs (NSAIDs), if tolerated; and antibiotics, if infection is believed to be the cause.

## Lateral epicondylitis (tennis elbow)

Lateral epicondylitis is inflammation and pain on the lateral aspect of the elbow at the insertion of the extensor tendons. It affects up to 50% of tennis players.

### Causes

The inflammation and irritation are caused by overuse of the hand and wrist extensors.

### Clinical features

The clinical features of lateral epicondylitis are:
- pain, which is worse with resisted extension and gripping
- point tenderness at the insertion of extensor carpi radialis brevis

### Investigations

The diagnosis is usually made on the history and clinical examination. If there is any doubt, anteroposterior and lateral radiographs are obtained, as well as an MRI to assess the soft tissues if the diagnosis remains uncertain.

### Management

Conservative management is most common. This consists of NSAIDs, support for the arm (counter-force strapping or bracing) and cessation of aggravating activities. Physiotherapy should be started. Consider steroid injection: this has limited benefit but should be considered before surgery is undertaken. Repeated steroid injection should be avoided. If the condition has become chronic, having continued for > 12 months, operative release and debridement are considered.

## Medial epicondylitis (golfer's elbow)

This condition is similar to lateral epicondylitis, except that it affects the common flexor origin. Pain is elicited with resisted flexion and on palpation of the medial epicondyle. It is less common than lateral epicondylitis; the diagnosis is clinical. The investigations are the same as those for lateral epicondylitis. The treatment regime is much the same as for lateral epicondylitis: rest, activity modification, NSAIDs and physiotherapy. Hydrocortisone injection may be tried (but avoid repeated hydrocortisone injection). If non-operative treatment fails then common flexor origin release is considered as the surgical option.

# Wrist and hand

Together, the many small bones and joints of the wrist and hand form a complex system that confers the ability to practise fine motor skills and carry out a wide range of movements.

## 6.1 Clinical scenario

### Wrist injury

#### Background

A 78-year-old man slipped while shopping, and fell on to an outstretched right hand. He felt an immediate pain in the wrist, and its range of movement is now very restricted. There is a large amount of swelling, and the injury continues to cause significant pain.

#### History

The patient has hypertension but is otherwise well. He is right-hand dominant. He lives alone and is very active, walking his dog at least once a day.

#### Examination

There is an obviously deformity at the wrist, but distally the hand is neurovascularly intact. The injury is closed, with only a minor superficial graze on the palm. The elbow and shoulder are fully examined, but no further injuries are identified.

#### Differential diagnosis

Possible injuries are:
- fracture of the distal radius or ulna
- carpal bone fracture or dislocation
- wrist dislocation

In a patient of this age group presenting with this mechanism of injury and examination findings, the most likely diagnosis is a distal radius fracture.

## Investigations

Posterioranterior and lateral radiographs of the wrist show a dorsally angulated fracture of the right distal radius, confirming what was suspected in the differential diagnosis. In the emergency department, the wrist is reduced into a satisfactory position and placed in a cast.

The patient is advised to use regular analgesia and keep the wrist elevated whenever possible. An appointment is made for visit to the fracture clinic in a week's time for reassessment and repeat imaging to ensure that the position of the wrist has been maintained.

---

## 6.2 Anatomy

The wrist and hand contain 27 bones, including the eight carpal bones (**Figure 6.1**). The distal row of carpal bones articulate with the metacarpal bones at the carpometacarpal joints. The metacarpal joints articulate with the phalanges at the metacarpophalangeal joints. The proximal interphalangeal joints are the hinge joints between the proximal and middle phalanges; the distal interphalangeal joints are the hinge joints between the middle and distal phalanges (**Figure 6.2**).

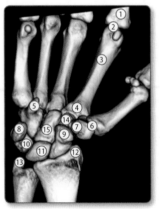

**Figure 6.1** 3D rendered CT image of the bones of the anterior wrist and hand ① Proximal phalanx, ② 2nd metacarpophalangeal joint, ③ 2nd metacarpal, ④ base of 2nd metacarpal, ⑤ hook of hamate, ⑥ 1st carpometacarpal joint, ⑦ trapezium, ⑧ pisiform, ⑨ scaphoid tubercle, ⑩ triquetrum (floor of carpal tunnel), ⑪ lunate (floor of carpal tunnel), ⑫ radial styloid process, ⑬ ulnar styloid process, ⑭ trapezoid, ⑮ capitate.

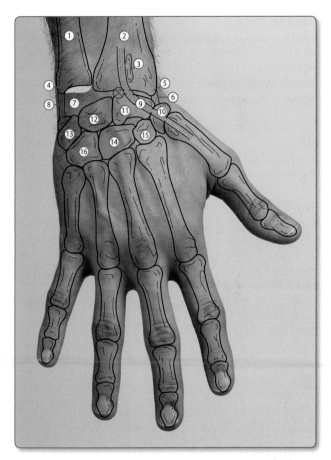

**Figure 6.2** Osteology and ligaments of the posterior wrist and hand. ① Ulna, ② radius, ③ dorsal radial (Lister's) tubercle, ④ ulna styloid process, ⑤ radial styloid process, ⑥ radial collateral ligament, ⑦ articular disc (triangular fibrocartilage), ⑧ ulna collateral ligament, ⑨ tendon of extensor pollicis longus, ⑩ trapezium, ⑪ scaphoid, ⑫ lunate, ⑬ triquetrum, capitate ⑭, trapezoid ⑮, hamate ⑯. ⊗ wrist injection/aspiration site.

## Vascular supply

Vascular supply is from the radial and ulnar arteries.

## Innervation

Motor and sensory supply is via the radial, ulnar and medial nerves. The sensory distribution is shown in **Figure 6.3**.

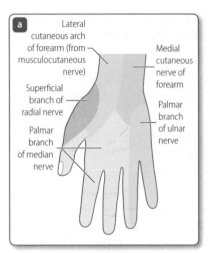

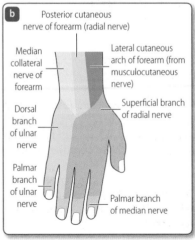

**Figure 6.3** Sensory distribution of the wrist and hand. (a) Anterior. (b) Posterior.

### Surface anatomy

Many joints of the wrist and hand are easily identifiable by their associated skin creases (**Figures 6.2** and **6.4**). The distal radius, ulnar styloid processes and carpal bones can be palpated.

---

## 6.3 Examination

### Key signs

Key signs to assess for include deformity, swelling, and the presence of any open wounds or neurovascular deficits.

### Examination sequence

Examination follows a system of 'Look, feel and move', and test of function, starting proximally and moving distally.

### Look

- Carry out an overall inspection for swelling and bruising
- Are there any obvious deformities of the wrist or fingers?
- Is there any obvious muscle wasting?

### Feel

- Palpate for bony tenderness
- Palpate for joint tenderness
- Palpate the distal radioulnar joint to assess stability
- Palpate the thenar and hypothenar eminences for muscle wasting and spasms

### Move

- Test for wrist movement: composite flexion/extension, abduction/adduction and pronation/supination (**Figure 6.5, 6.6** and **6.7**)
- Test for full range of movement of the metacarpophalangeal, proximal interphalangeal and distal interphalangeal joints
- Carry out functional tests of the hand, including Phalen's test (**Figure 6.8**) for key, pinch, precision and power grip

### Function

- Assess the patient's fine motor skills, grip and dexterity
- Ask the patient about their ability to eat, write and open doors
- Assess their sensitivity to touch

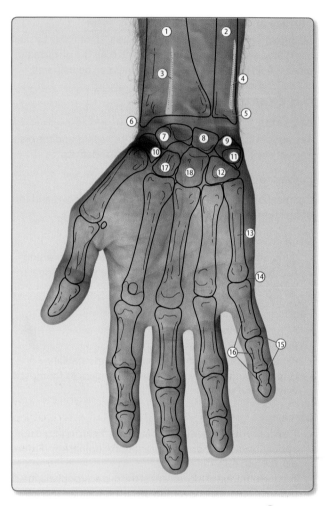

**Figure 6.4** Osteology and ligaments of the anterior wrist and hand. ① Radius, ② ulna, ③ line of flexor carpi radialis tendon, ④ line of flexor carpi ulnaris tendon, ⑤ ulna styloid process, ⑥ radial styloid process, ⑦ scaphoid tubercle, ⑧ lunate, ⑨ triquetrum, ⑩ trapezium tubercle, ⑪ pisiform, ⑫ hook of hamate, ⑬ metacarpal bones, ⑭ metacarpophalangeal joint, ⑮ interphalangeal joints (proximal and distal), ⑯ phalangeal bones (proximal, middle and distal), ⑰ trapezoid, ⑱ capitate.

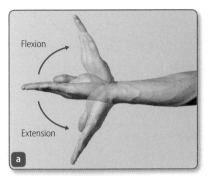

**Figure 6.5** Wrist movements. (a) Extension/flexion (70–75°). (b) Abduction/adduction.

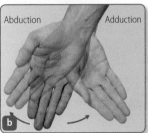

## 6.4 Mid-shaft fractures of the forearm

Mid-shaft fractures of the forearm are associated with distal radioulnar joint injuries (DRUJ), Galeazzi fractures or radial head dislocation/instability, and Monteggia fractures. It is important, therefore, to examine both the wrist and elbow joints in these patients. Mid-shaft fractures of the forearm have the second highest ratio of open:closed fracture of any bone, second to the tibia.

### Epidemiology
This type of fracture is more common in men than women.

### Causes
The usual cause is a direct blow, fall or sporting injury.

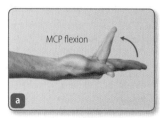

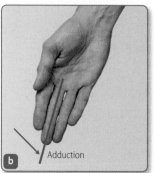

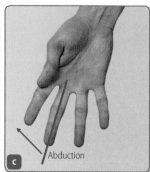

**Figure 6.6** Hand movements. (a) MCP flexion (90°). (b) Finger adduction. (c) Finger abduction.

### Clinical features

The patient is in pain, and their forearm appears swollen and bruised. There may be an obvious deformity.

Neurovascular status is fully assessed, and the results are documented. Monitoring for compartment syndrome is essential, because it is associated with these fractures and leads to irreversible muscle and nerve damage. The elbow, wrist and shoulder are also assessed to exclude additional injuries.

### Investigations

AP and lateral radiographs of the forearm are obtained. If there is any clinical concern of an associated DRUJ or elbow injury, further radiographs of the elbow and wrist are carried out.

### Management

Most mid-shaft forearm fractures are treated surgically to stabilise the bone and reduce the risk of mal- or non-union.

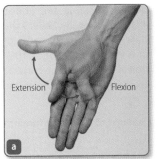

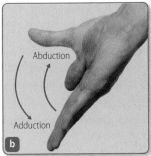

Extension        Flexion

Abduction

Adduction

a

b

**Figure 6.7** Thumb movements. (a) Extension/flexion. (b) Adduction/abduction. (c) Thumb opposition (anterior view).

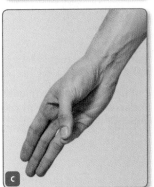

c

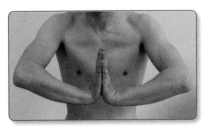

**Figure 6.8** Prayer sign.

**Conservative management** A single-bone fracture of the forearm may be managed conservatively if angulation is < 10°. If patients are unsuitable candidates for surgery, a well-moulded cast and follow-up in the fracture clinic are sufficient.

**Surgical management** All displaced, unstable, both-bone fractures of the forearm are managed surgically, unless the patient is an unsuitable candidate for surgery. In cases of individual radial or ulnar fractures with angulation > 10%, surgical fixation is required. Surgical management consists of anatomical reduction and fixation, usually with a plate and screws.

**Complications** Potential complications of mid-shaft forearm fractures are:

- malunion or non-union
- infection
- neurovascular damage
- refracture

## 6.5 Distal radius fractures

Distal radius fractures are one of the most common injuries seen in orthopaedics. They are classified according to the direction of angulation and whether or not there is articular involvement (**Table 6.1**).

### Epidemiology

Fractures of the distal radius occur in a bimodal distribution. The incidence peaks in women over 50 years of age.

| Eponymous name | Description |
|---|---|
| Colles fracture | Fracture of the distal radius, with dorsal angulation; extra-articular |
| Smith fracture | Fracture of the distal radius, with volar angulation (inherently more unstable); extra-articular |
| Barton fracture | Fracture of the distal radius, with involvement of the articular surface, either the dorsal or volar aspect |
| Chauffeur's fracture | Intra-articular radial styloid fracture |

**Table 6.1** Classification of fractures of the distal radius.

## Causes

In younger patients, these fractures are caused by high-energy injuries. In older patients, simple falls tend to be the mechanism of injury.

## Clinical features

Pain and a marked reduction in range of movement, as well as swelling and bruising, are all likely to be present. It is important to check that the injury is closed and the limb neurovascularly intact, because any open injury or neurovascular compromise requires urgent senior assessment and management.

## Investigations

AP or PA and lateral radiographs of the wrist are required (**Figures 6.9** and **6.10**). CT is needed if the fracture pattern cannot be fully assessed using radiographs.

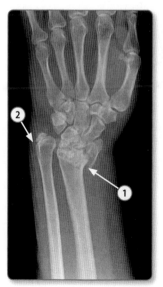

**Figure 6.9** Posteroanterior radiograph of the wrist, showing a comminuted shortened fracture of the distal radius ① and ulnar styloid ②. The fracture of the radius is intra-articular.

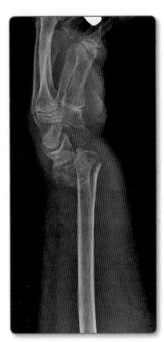

**Figure 6.10** Lateral radiograph of the wrist, showing an 'off-ended' fracture of the distal radius. The fracture is also dorsally angulated and shortened ('bayonetted').

Patients may be referred for measurement of bone density (by DEXA scan). This particularly useful if they are post-menopausal women in whom osteoporosis is suspected.

## Management

The majority of distal radius fractures, particularly in the elderly, are managed non-operatively. The aims of treatment are to reduce the fracture and achieve articular congruency.

**Conservative management**   The fracture can be managed with application of a cast and follow-up in the fracture clinic if there is < 5 mm of shortening and < 5° of angulation. A cast is also adequate treatment if the patient is an unsuitable candidate for surgery.

When applying a cast, reduction can be attempted with traction and manipulation. Appropriate analgesia is required for this procedure, with either a haematoma or Bier block, or anaesthetic gas (e.g. Entonox).

**Surgical management**  Surgical management is indicated if:
- the fracture is unstable, i.e. there is angulation (> 5°) or shortening (> 5 mm)
- the fracture is comminuted
- there is disruption of the joint surface

Fixation is achieved with the use of a plate and screws (**Figure 6.11**).

**Complications**  All fractures of the distal radius are associated with chronic swelling and stiffness, which lasts for up

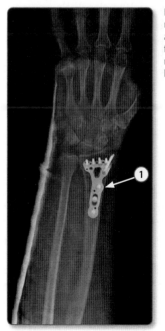

**Figure 6.11** Posteroanterior radiograph of a wrist showing a locking plate ① fixation of a fracture of the distal radius. Excellent reduction of the articular surface and length has been achieved.

to 18 months. Occasionally, this stiffness and swelling is permanent.

In malreduced fractures, permanent bony deformity is likely, but this is usually not troublesome. Fractures healed in dorsal angulation cause loss of grip strength, and patients have difficulty palmar flexing the wrist. All malreduced fractures result in loss of pronation or supination at the wrist, which may impair a patient's ability to carry out their daily activities.

Clinically troublesome osteoarthritis is rare, but it can occur in cases of intra-articular fracture. Complex regional pain syndrome type 1 can develop after fracture of the distal radius. Its signs and symptoms include pain in a non-anatomical distribution, stiffness and a change of colour in the affected limb.

## 6.6 Distal radioulnar joint injuries

The distal radioulnar joint (DRUJ) is the articulation of the sigmoid notch of the distal radius with the ulnar head (**Figure 6.12**). The main soft tissue components are the triangular fibrocartilage complex and the radioulnar ligament. The interosseous membrane also stabilises this joint complex.

### Epidemiology

DRUJ injuries occur most frequently in younger patients who sustain high-energy wrist injuries.

### Causes

DRUJ injuries can occur in isolation, but are commonly associated with fractures of the distal radius. For example:

- The DRUJ is dislocated in cases of fracture of the distal third of the radial shaft with disruption of the DRUJ (Galeazzi fracture).

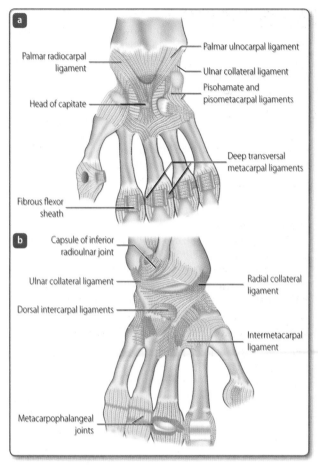

**Figure 6.12** Ligaments of the distal radioulnar joint. (a) Anterior. (b) Posterior.

- Dislocation of the DRUJ is found in combination with comminuted radial head fracture (Essex-Lopresti fracture); the fracture propagates through the intraosseous membrane. Both of these injuries are very unstable.

### Clinical features

Pain, instability, reduced range of movement and reduced grip strength are all signs of distal radioulnar joint injury. It should be considered in all wrist injuries, because it is easily overlooked. On examination, the patient has dorsal or ulnar wrist pain, and squeezing the joint provokes pain. There may also be clicking on movement of the joint.

### Investigations

Anteroposterior and lateral radiographs show widening of the distal radioulnar joint. They also show any dorsal displacement. MRI is indicated if a tear to the triangular fibrocartilage is suspected.

### Management

DRUJ injuries are usually treated non-operatively, with 4 weeks of immobilisation. A grossly unstable distal radioulnar joint requires stabilisation with Kirschner wires. If the injury is associated with a fracture, open reduction and internal fixation is required.

Galeazzi fractures are treated with open reduction and internal fixation of the distal radius, as well as pinning of the distal radioulnar joint.

**Complications** Common complications include pain and stiffness. DRUJ injuries, particularly if not recognised, lead to chronic instability and arthritis.

## 6.7 Scaphoid fractures

The scaphoid sits on the radial side of the carpus, and is the largest of the bones of the proximal row. It forms the floor of the anatomical snuffbox, within which it can be palpated (**Figure 6.13**).

The scaphoid receives its blood supply from the lateral and distal branches of the radial artery. Fractures of the waist or proximal third depend on union of the fracture for revascularisation. Non-unions result in loss of blood supply to the

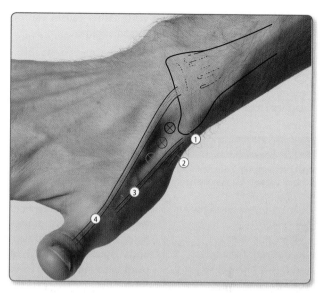

**Figure 6.13** Borders and bones of the anatomical snuffbox. ① Radial styloid process, ② abductor pollicis longus tendon, ③ extensor pollicis brevis tendon, ④ extensor pollicis longus tendon, ⊗ scaphoid, ⊗ trapezium, ⊗ base of 1st metacarpal.

proximal pole, so there is a high risk of avascular necrosis in such cases.

### Epidemiology

The scaphoid is the most commonly fractured carpal bone (50–80% of all carpal bone fractures). Most scaphoid fractures are through the waist of the scaphoid (>50% of cases). About 25% of cases are through the proximal pole and the remainder through the distal pole.

### Causes

The most common cause of a scaphoid fracture is a fall on to an outstretched hand, which leads to loading across a hyperextended and radially deviated wrist. Other causes can be 'kickback', for example when starting an engine.

## Clinical features

Patients present with wrist pain and swelling, and have tenderness in the anatomical snuffbox or over the scaphoid tubercle. Scaphoid fractures cause pain on resisted pronation.

### Clinical insight

Scaphoid views are four radiographs that optimise visualisation of the scaphoid specifically:

- posteroanterior view of the wrist, with ulnar deviation
- lateral view of the wrist
- oblique view of the wrist
- scaphoid view (20–30° tube angle)

The scaphoid view provides an elongated image of the scaphoid that may show a fracture not apparent on any other view.

## Investigations

Posteroanterior and lateral radiographs of the wrist are usually the first images requested. If a scaphoid fracture is suspected, specific scaphoid views (four different projections) are obtained to aid diagnosis (**Figure 6.14**). In 25% of cases, initial radiographs fail to show a fracture. However, if a fracture is suspected clinically, the patient is immobilised and radiography repeated after 1–2 weeks.

The most sensitive investigation for diagnosis of acute scaphoid fractures is MRI. CT may also be used, but it is not as effective acutely. It is more beneficial at a later stage to assess union.

## Management

Management of scaphoid fractures varies; always check the local department protocol.

**Conservative management** If a scaphoid injury is suspected but no fracture is apparent on radiography, management consists of immobilisation in a wrist splint with a thumb extension or in a scaphoid cast. After 2 weeks, further radiographs are obtained for reassessment. If evidence of a fracture is found, the wrist remains immobilised in a scaphoid plaster for up to 4 months, or until there is evidence of union, with close monitoring to ensure that avascular necrosis does not develop and the fracture achieves full union.

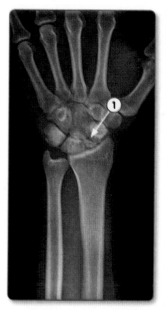

**Figure 6.14** Posteroanterior radiograph showing a transverse fracture ① through the waist of the scaphoid.

Stable, non-displaced fractures are managed by immobilisation in a scaphoid cast. Scaphoid casts hold the wrist in slight dorsiflexion and extend along the thumb.

**Surgical management** This is indicated for:

- proximal pole fractures
- fractures of the waist with > 1 mm of displacement
- non-union
- unstable or angulated fractures

Surgery is carried out either open or closed with percutaneous screws, depending on surgical preference and the type of fracture. Bone grafting is more commonly required in non-unions or chronic injuries.

**Complications** Common complications are:

- avascular necrosis (apparent on radiographs by 1–2 months)
- non-union, delayed union or malunion
- arthritis

## 6.8 Lunate and perilunate dislocations

The lunate is normally firmly attached by ligaments to the distal radius. It has been called the 'carpal keystone', because of its key contribution to the stability of the wrist.

In a lunate dislocation, the lunate dislocates in the volar or dorsal direction but the carpus remains aligned

In a perilunate dislocation, the lunate stays in position and the carpus dislocates (**Figures 6.15** and **6.16**)

A sequence of progressive perilunate instability occurs as the injury spreads. This is described by the Mayfield classification (**Table 6.2**).

Failure to identify these injuries can leave the patient with an extremely poor functional outcome. In cases of doubt, the opinion of a senior colleague must be sought.

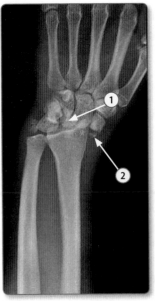

**Figure 6.15** Anteroposterior radiograph of the wrist, showing perilunate dislocation. The carpus has dislocated around the lunate ①. It has deviated radially. An associated scaphoid fracture ② is visible. There is clear abnormality, but this image is difficult to interpret.

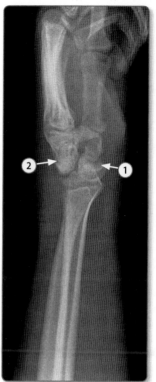

**Figure 6.16** Lateral radiograph of the same wrist shown in Figure 6.12. This image is easier to interpret than the anteroposterior radiograph. It confirms dorsal dislocation of the carpus ② around the lunate ①, which has remained in its usual position. The lunate has an empty concavity.

| Stage | Description |
|-------|-------------|
| I | Disruption of scapholunate joint |
| II | Disruption of lunocapitate joint |
| III | Disruption of lunotriquetral joint |
| IV | Lunate dislocation |

**Table 6.2** Mayfield classification of lunate dislocations.

## Epidemiology

Lunate and perilunate dislocations are rare, but often missed. Dislocations of the lunate are the most common of all carpal dislocations, and must be considered when the wrist is significantly swollen and the mechanism of injury is likely to cause lunate dislocation. These injuries can happen at any age, but are more common in 18–50 year olds.

## Causes

The mechanism of injury is application of a load to the extended wrist. It is a high-energy injury.

## Clinical features

Patients present with wrist swelling and pain. They have tenderness on palpation just distal to the dorsal tubercle of the radius (Lister's tubercle). They may also have median nerve symptoms.

## Investigations

Posteroanterior and lateral radiographs of the wrist are obtained. It is important to assess Gilula's arcs on the posteroanterior radiograph. Any disruption indicates ligamentous instability, dislocation or fracture (**Figure 6.17**).

On the posteroanterior radiograph, the lunate and capitate may overlap, or the lunate may appear triangular rather than squarish in contour, in cases of lunate or perilunate dislocation.

It is much easier to diagnose these injuries on the lateral radiograph. There is disruption of the normal arrangement, i.e. the radius, lunate and capitate in a straight line, and the capitate sitting in the concavity of the lunate.

- In lunate dislocations, the concavity of the lunate is empty, and the radius and capitate remain in a straight line
- In perilunate dislocations, the concavity is empty and the radius and lunate remain in a straight line; the capitate lies dorsally, out of line (see **Figure 6.16**)

On all views, it is important to look for other associated fractures of the carpal bones. Perilunate dislocations are commonly associated with scaphoid fractures.

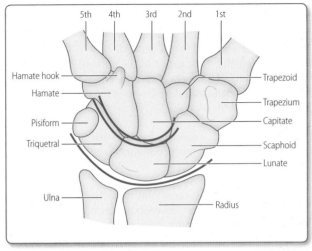

**Figure 6.17** Gilula's arcs are used to assess carpal alignment on the PA radiograph.

A CT scan is often useful to further assess the pattern of injury.

## Management

All lunate and perilunate dislocations require urgent closed reduction and splinting. Immediate surgery is indicated if the dislocation cannot be reduced closed, or if there is any sign of median nerve compression. Closed reduction is followed by open reduction and soft tissue reconstruction at a later date.

If the injury is chronic, referral to a hand or upper limb specialist is required for possible carpectomy or arthrodesis. Physiotherapy is needed if there is residual stiffness.

**Complications**  Common complications are:

- median nerve neuropathy
- chronic instability
- osteoarthritis
- avascular necrosis

## 6.9 Metacarpal fractures

Metacarpal fractures are classified as head, neck and shaft fractures. Management varies depending on which metacarpal is affected and the location of the fracture. These injuries are common hand fractures, seen regularly in the emergency department and fracture clinics.

### Epidemiology

Metacarpal fractures, especially fractures of the 5th metacarpal neck (**Figure 6.18**), are most commonly seen in young men.

### Causes

These fractures are most commonly caused by direct trauma to the hand, for example from delivering a punch (boxer's fracture), crush injury or a road traffic accident (in which case multiple hand fractures are likely). A high percentage of these fractures are work-related injuries.

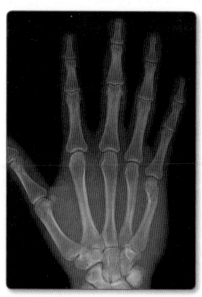

**Figure 6.18**
Anteroposterior radiograph of the hand, showing a fracture of the 5th metacarpal neck.

## Clinical features

Patients present with a painful, swollen hand. Grazes or other soft tissue injuries are likely to be present. Compartment syndrome is a risk, particularly in cases of crush injury or multiple hand fractures. However, it is a rare complication of metacarpal fractures.

The finger is assessed for shortening, angulation and rotational deformity, but this is sometimes difficult because of the swelling. Both hands are examined with the metacarpophalangeals and interphalangeal joints flexed. All fingers should point to the scaphoid tubercle, and all the nails should align in the same plane. Asymmetry indicates deformity. The hands are compared and differences between them noted.

Distal neurological and vascular status are assessed.

## Investigations

Anteroposterior, oblique and lateral radiographs of the hand are obtained. CT is necessary if the injury is a very complex and comminuted fracture of the metacarpal head.

Dislocation requires accurate reduction; if missed or not treated properly they have a poor prognosis. Dislocation is more common in the carpometacarpal joint of the index and little fingers. A true lateral radiograph shows dislocation or subluxation at the carpometacarpal joint in cases of dislocation.

## Management

Apart from the fracture pattern, associated neurovascular injury and whether the fracture is open or closed, other points that help determine whether or not to operate include:

- hand dominance
- occupation
- age
- comorbidities
- mechanism of injury

Non-displaced transverse or longitudinal fractures are generally stable. Displaced fractures and spiral fractures, and some oblique fractures, are more likely to be unstable.

**Conservative management** Non-operative management is used if the fracture is closed and stable, and there is minimal shortening (< 2–5 mm), acceptable angulation of both neck and shaft (**Table 6.3**) and no rotational deformity. The hand is immobilised in a back slab or plaster with a finger extension. Neighbour strapping, i.e. strapping the injured finger to an adjacent finger, often suffices. The fracture first requires reduction or manipulation following administration of adequate analgesia.

**Surgical management** Operative treatment is indicated for intra-articular fractures, rotational deformity, significant shaft or neck angulation (see **Table 6.3**), open fractures, multiple metacarpal fractures and fractures associated with tendon injury. Fractures to the border digit metacarpal shafts are less stable than non-border digits, therefore surgery is often indicated.

All carpometacarpal subluxations and dislocations require reduction and fixation. This is carried out by open reduction and internal fixation with percutaneous pinning (Kirschner wires) or plating, or external fixation (if the soft tissues are particularly swollen).

To reduce stiffness, the patient must start mobilising the hand by at least 4 weeks

## Clinical insight

The patient may have a 'fight bite'. If the patient has an open wound overlying the metacarpophalangeal joint or another joint in the hand, the possibility of a bite injury is considered.

In many cases, the patient has punched another person in the mouth, resulting in laceration by a tooth. The puncture is effectively a bite. Because these wounds are caused by teeth, there is a significant risk of contamination by oral flora. Washout, debridement and oral antibiotics are required. It is not unusual for teeth to be found in these wounds on exploration.

| Metacarpal | Acceptable shaft angle (°) | Acceptable neck angle (°) |
| --- | --- | --- |
| Index and middle | 10–20 | 10–15 |
| Ring | 30 | 30–40 |
| Little | 40 | 50–60 |

Table 6.3 Acceptable angulation in metacarpal fractures.

after injury. Postoperative physiotherapy and occupational therapy are crucial.

**Complications**   The most common complications of metacarpal fractures are:

- reduced range of movement
- stiffness
- deformity
- malunion

## 6.10 Phalangeal fractures

Phalangeal fractures are classified as distal, middle and proximal phalanx fractures. Dislocations of the proximal and distal interphalangeal joints are also common and can easily be missed.

### Epidemiology

Phalangeal fractures are the most common bony injury and the distal phalanx is the most commonly fractured bone in the hand.

### Causes

The most common cause in different age groups are:

- sport injuries in young adults
- trauma and injuries from machinery in people aged 35–70 years
- falls in the elderly

### Clinical features

Patients present with pain, deformity and reduced range of movement. Rotational deformity is assessed. Wounds or associated nail bed injuries may be present (see page 183). The extensor and flexor tendons are assessed, and the neurovascular status of the finger is documented.

### Investigations

Anteroposterior and lateral radiographs of the finger and hand are obtained to exclude other bony injuries or dislocations (**Figure 6.19**). All radiographs must be examined thoroughly, because small avulsion fracture at the margins of joints indicate

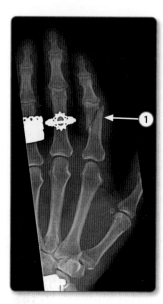

**Figure 6.19** Anteroposterior radiograph of the hand, showing an extra-articular spiral fracture to the proximal phalanx of the index finger ①.

more serious soft tissue injuries and have important functional implications.

## Management

The management varies on whether the proximal, middle or distal phalanx is injured, the fracture configuration, amount of angulation, and whether the fracture is open or closed or has associated injuries.

**Conservative management**  A fracture that is reducible, extra-articular and minimally displaced (< 10° of angulation or < 2 mm shortening) and has no rotational deformity is treated conservatively with immobilisation by neighbour strapping for 3–4 weeks. A ring block using local anaesthetic is required for reduction.

An isolated dislocation is reduced under ring block anaesthesia, and if stable, the patient should be able to start active movement immediately. If the dislocation is unstable, immobilisation for about 3 weeks is required.

**Surgical management**  A fracture that is irreducible, intra-articular or unstable (> 10° of angulation or > 2 mm shortening) or has a rotational deformity usually requires manipulation under anaesthesia and Kirschner wire stabilisation or open reduction and internal fixation. The treatment is similar for fractures of the proximal and middle phalanx.

Distal fractures sometimes require nail bed repair (see page 183). Dislocations and very unstable reductions require open reduction and either Kirschner wire stabilisation or screw fixation (**Figure 6.20**).

**Complications**  Common complications are:
- stiffness

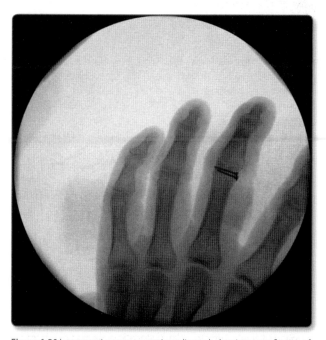

**Figure 6.20** Intraoperative anteroposterior radiograph showing screw fixation of a condylar fracture of the proximal phalanx of the middle finger.

- reduced range of movement
- malunion, non-union or delayed union
- osteoarthritis and possible need for arthrodesis in later life

## 6.11 Base-of-thumb fractures

The carpometacarpal joint at the base of the thumb is multifunctional. It can adduct, abduct, oppose and circumduct.

These injuries are either extra-articular or intra-articular. There are two main types of intra-articular fracture:

- Rolando fractures, comminuted intra-articular fractures (commonly called Y fractures) (**Figure 6.21**)
- Bennett fractures, two-part intra-articular fractures (**Figure 6.22**)

The abductor pollicis longus, adductor pollicis and extensor pollicis longus are the muscles that can deform and displace thumb fractures.

### Epidemiology
Most fractures of the thumb involve the base. Bennett fractures are the most common.

### Causes
Base-of-thumb fractures are caused by application of an axial force to the thumb, or forced abduction.

### Clinical features
Patients present with pain and swelling of the thumb and hand.

### Investigations
Anteroposterior, lateral and oblique radiographs are required to confirm the bony injury. A CT scan is performed if further anatomical information is needed.

### Management
**Conservative management** Most extra-articular fractures with minimal displacement and < 30° of angulation are treated non-operatively with immobilisation in a thumb spica splint. For non-displaced Bennett fractures, the thumb can be put

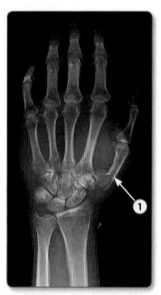

**Figure 6.21** Anteroposterior radiograph showing a Rolando fracture of the base of the thumb ①. The inverted T pattern is characteristic.

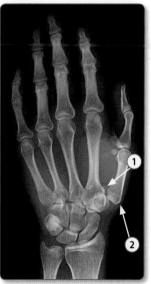

**Figure 6.22** Anteroposterior radiograph of the hand, showing a Bennett fracture of the base of the thumb. The small fracture fragment ① has remained in position, allowing the metacarpal ② to sublux.

### Clinical insight

Skier's thumb (fall on to a hand holding a ski pole) and gamekeeper's thumb (caused by movement used to kill rabbits) are the rupture or severe stretching, respectively, of the ulnar collateral ligament to the thumb. If the metacarpophalangeal joint opens more than 30° on abduction, there is likely to be a complete rupture. This type of injury often requires surgery because of the possibility of a Stener lesion, which is characterised by displacement of the avulsed bone resulting in it sitting above the adductor aponeurosis, thereby blocking its reduction and precluding healing.

If skier's thumb or gamekeeper's thumb goes unrecognised and untreated, the joint may sublux, leading to permanent disability. An associated avulsion fracture may be visible on the radiograph, but it appears normal in most cases.

into a cast or thumb splint and immobilised.

Dislocations are reduced closed. Conservative management is best for severely comminuted Rolando fractures, but it is important to get the patient moving early to prevent the stiffness associated with immobilisation.

**Surgical management** Extra-articular fractures require surgical management if there is > 30° of angulation. They are held by Kirschner wires, or open reduction and internal fixation is carried out.

If there is significant displacement of a Bennett fracture, or the fracture moves in the cast, open reduction and internal fixation is indicated (**Figure 6.23**). A screw is used to hold the fracture.

For Rolando fractures, open reduction and internal fixation is an option. However, external fixation is considered if there is significant swelling and severe comminution.

**Complications**  Associated complications are:

- osteoarthritis
- stiffness

## 6.12 Tendon (flexor and extensor) injuries of the wrist and hand

Tendon injuries of the hand are classified as either flexor or extensor. They are further described by the location of injury: flexor tendon injuries are classified into five zones (see **Figure 6.25**) and extensor tendon injuries into eight zones.

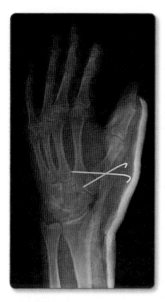

**Figure 6.23** Posteroanterior radiograph showing Kirschner wire fixation of a Bennett fracture, with reduction of the fracture and good alignment of the thumb.

## Epidemiology

Traumatic injuries to tendons are more common in younger patients. Certain comorbidities are associated with tendon rupture, such as rheumatoid arthritis and extensor tendon rupture.

## Causes

Tendon injuries are caused by direct trauma, lacerations or repetitive overuse.

## Clinical features

Patients present with pain, possible wounds and the inability to actively flex or extend at a joint. A thorough examination is required to determine the specific tendon injured. The patient is also assessed for any other neurovascular injuries. Lacerations and punctures are looked for; any penetrating injury may cause laceration of a tendon.

## Clinical insight

Mallet finger (**Figure 6.24**) is a common hand injury caused by forced flexion of an extended finger leading to disruption of the extensor tendon. It is associated with fracture of the dorsal lip of the distal phalanx. The patient is unable to fully extend the distal interphalangeal joint.

If there is no bony injury, the DIP joint of the finger is splinted in extension in a mallet splint for 6–8 weeks. If there is a significant avulsion fragment, Kirschner wires are required to maintain reduction and stabilise the fracture.

### Investigations

Anteroposterior and lateral radiographs of the finger are obtained to rule out any bony avulsion fractures and the presence of a foreign body (e.g. glass). In cases of doubt, US can be used to confirm partial or complete rupture.

### Management

The zone of injury guides splinting and surgical repair options as well as prognosis (**Figure 6.25**).

Zone 2 flexor tendon lacerations require great care to restore normal anatomy, as both deep and superficial tendons pass through here. The tendons must be repaired so that they continue to pass freely over one another. When repairing extensor tendons, care is required to restore the slips over the metacarpophalangeal and proximal interphalangeal joint, thereby facilitating normal movement.

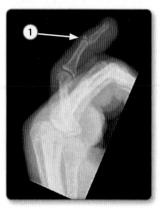

**Figure 6.24** Lateral radiograph of the finger, showing bony mallet avulsion ① to the terminal phalanx.

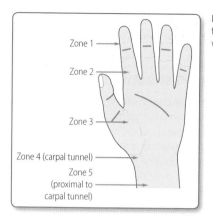

**Figure 6.25** Zones of flexor tendon injury in the wrist and hand.

Zone 1

Zone 2

Zone 3

Zone 4 (carpal tunnel)

Zone 5 (proximal to carpal tunnel)

**Conservative management** Tendon injuries with < 50% of the tendon width in the extensor tendons and with extension and flexion capability can be managed conservatively. Complete immobilisation in a splint for 6 weeks is followed by further splinting for 4–6 weeks while starting joint motion. The type of splinting depends on whether it is a flexor tendon or extensor tendon injury, and the level of injury.

Rehabilitation is achieved by physiotherapy and occupational therapy to optimise movement. Most partial lacerations of flexor tendons require exploration and surgical repair.

**Surgical management** Tendon repair is indicated for:
- open wounds requiring closure;
- injuries involving > 50% tendon width in extensor tendons and flexor tendons;
- injuries with associated displaced bony avulsion fractures or phalanx fractures.

Tendon reconstruction is required if repair is not possible, as either a one- or two-stage procedure using grafts. Splinting and intensive postoperative physiotherapy or occupational therapy are required.

**Complications** The most common complications are:
- rerupture

- stiffness as a consequence of adhesions
- finger deformity
- contractures

## 6.13 Flexor tendon sheath infection

The flexor tendons are contained within a synovial sheath running from the distal interphalangeal joint to the mid-palm and wrist. The function of the sheath is to protect and nourish the tendons. If it becomes infected, there is rapid loss of function of the hand and the potential for irreversible damage to the flexor tendons and the delicate structures around them. Therefore infection of the flexor tendon sheath is an orthopaedic emergency.

### Epidemiology
Any age group can be affected. Intravenous drug users and patients with diabetes are at increased risk.

### Causes
Flexor tendon sheath infection can be caused by direct trauma to the hand, or the fingers specifically, including superficial lacerations, penetration by splinters or thorns, and animal bites. Infection can also spread from septic joints. The most common causative organism is *Staphylococcus aureus*.

### Clinical insight

The four cardinal signs of flexor sheath infection, known as Kanavel signs, are:
- the finger is held in a flexed position
- fusiform swelling of the finger
- tenderness over the affected tendon
- pain on passive extension

### Clinical features
Patients present with pain in one of their fingers, spreading to the palm. The finger is swollen and warm, with erythema and reduced movement. Evidence of a wound, splinter, bite or similar is present.

### Investigations
Measurement of inflammatory markers is useful, so include full blood count, C-reactive protein and erythrocyte sedimentation rate when organising blood tests.

## Management

Flexor tendon sheath infections are an orthopaedic emergency, so an urgent review and referral to a senior colleague is required to plan further management.

**Conservative management**  If the patient presents early, treatment consists of elevation, use of IV antibiotics and close observation. If there is no improvement within 24 h, surgery is required.

**Surgical management**  Most patients require washout of the flexor tendon sheath and admission for administration of IV antibiotics.

**Complications**  Potential complications of infection of the flexor tendon sheath are:
- reduced flexion of finger
- stiffness
- recurrent infection

## 6.14 Nail bed injuries

These include nail bed lacerations, nail avulsions and subungual haematomas. There may also be associated fractures or dislocations of the distal phalanx. **Figure 6.26** shows the anatomy of the nail bed.

### Epidemiology

Nail bed injuries are very common hand injuries in children and adults.

### Causes

Injuries result from direct trauma to the fingertip:
- Crush injuries from heavy objects, for example paving slabs
- Injury from a door closing on the finger
- Workplace injuries, for example hammer or saw injuries

### Clinical features

The fingertip has a painful wound, with extensive injury and swelling. There is often subungual haematoma. The nail may

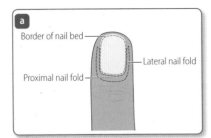

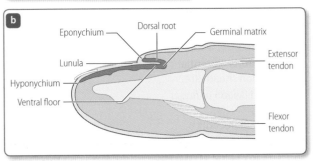

**Figure 6.26** Anatomy of the nail bed. (a) Top view. (b) Side view.

or may not be present. Given the mechanism of injury, there is usually an associated fracture of the terminal phalanx.

### Investigations
Anteroposterior and lateral radiographs of the finger are required to check for fractures.

### Management
Isolated, small subungual haematomas are drained by puncture with a sterile needle or electocautery. If severe (> 50% of the nail bed), the nail is removed for evacuation of the haematoma and subsequent repair of the nail bed. In adults, this is done under local digital ring block. Young children require general anaesthesia.

Any laceration with an underlying fracture requires nail removal and repair. The nail is removed, the wound washed out, the nail bed repaired with sutures, and normally either the old nail or a nail-shaped splint is used to protect the nail bed and splint the eponychial fold open to help the new nail grow. Antibiotics (IV in theatre and oral on discharge) and tetanus vaccine are administered.

Fractures of the distal phalanx require fixation, for example with Kirschner wire. Injuries with significant loss of pulp, nail bed and tissue occasionally require terminalisation; the patient should be warned of this, because these injuries can only be fully assessed after thorough washout, administration of anaesthetic and use of a tourniquet.

**Complications**   Common complications are:
- failure of the nail to regrow
- nail ridges
- hook nail
- loss of the fingertip

## 6.15 Paronychia

Paronychia is the commonest infection of the hand. Soft tissue inflammation of the lateral nail fold is most commonly caused by *S. aureus* infection. Paronychia is usually caused by nail biting, manicures or prolonged exposure to water and resultant breakdown of the skin, for example in gardeners and hairdressers. People with diabetes, psoriasis, eczema or on steroid treatment are at increased risk.

The patient presents with a painful, swollen, erythematous nail fold that has purulent discharge. In chronic cases, there are usually nail changes. These often settle with cleaning and use of oral antibiotics but occasionally require incision and drainage.

## 6.16 Other carpal fractures

### Triquetral fractures

The triquetrum is the most commonly fractured bone after the scaphoid. Triquetral fractures are commonly associated with ligamentous injuries. Patients typically have tenderness on the dorsal ulnar aspect of the wrist, and a painful range of wrist movement.

An oblique radiograph, along with anteroposterior and lateral radiographs, is required for better assessment. On the lateral radiograph, a small fragment lying posterior to the proximal row of the carpus invariably represents a fracture of the triquetrum. Non-displaced fractures are treated in a below-elbow cast for 6 weeks. Displaced fractures require open reduction and internal fixation.

## Pisiform fractures

This injury is rare. The pisiform is a sesamoid bone located in the flexor carpi ulnaris tendon. Patients present with ulnar-sided wrist pain and point tenderness after a direct blow to the volar aspect of the wrist or a fall on to an outstretched hand.

Pisiform fractures are usually associated with distal radial, triquetral or hamate fractures. They may be visualised on radiographs but are best seen by CT. Treatment is immobilisation, usually in a splint. If chronic pain persists or a non-union occurs, pisiformectomy is occasionally required at a later date.

## Hamate fractures

Fractures of the hamate are of the body of the bone or, more commonly, the hook. Generally, fractures of the body are caused by direct trauma or crush injuries to the hand. Hook-of-hamate fractures frequently result from trauma to the palm of the hand when it is struck by an object, and are therefore usually sporting injuries, for example from racquets, golf clubs or hockey sticks.

Patients present with pain and tenderness, typically over the hypothenar eminence and hamate. They may have decreased grip strength and paraesthesia in the ulnar nerve distribution, as a consequence of nerve compression. Radiography and CT are recommended. The wrist is immobilised, usually in a splint, for 4–6 weeks. Occasionally, open reduction and internal fixation or excision of the hamate is required. If nerve injury is suspected, surgical exploration is required.

# chapter 7

# Hip

The hip is a synovial ball and socket joint in which the femur articulates with the acetabulum. It is unusual because it is very stable yet allows a large range of motion.

The main role of the hip is to support the weight of the body, both in stance and motion. Hip injury can therefore be debilitating and cause long-lasting impairment of mobility. The main mechanisms of hip joint injury are falls in the elderly and high-energy injuries in younger patients. Patients generally present with pain and an inability to mobilise or weight-bear.

## 7.1 Clinical scenario

### Hip pain

#### Background

An 84-year-old woman got up to visit the toilet in the middle of the night. On standing up from the toilet she slipped, landing on her left side. She was unable to get up. Her daughter found her on the floor the next morning. An ambulance was called.

#### History

The patient has a past medical history of hypertension, angina, atrial fibrillation and osteoporosis. Her regular medications include amlodipine, lisinopril, a glyceryl trinitrate spray, warfarin and simvastatin. A cleaner does her housework once a week, and she walks with a stick, but otherwise her health conditions do not limit her activities of daily living. She lives alone.

#### Examination

Inspection finds bruising over the left greater trochanter. The left leg is shortened and externally rotated, and the patient is unable to lift it. Considerable pain is elicited on any attempted passive movement. No neurovascular deficit is noted.

### Differential diagnosis

Possible injuries are:

- fractured neck of femur
- pubic ramus fracture
- pelvic fracture
- soft tissue injury
- exacerbation of osteoarthritis of the hip

The most common diagnosis in elderly patients presenting to the emergency department after a fall and unable to weight bear is a fractured neck of femur.

### Investigations

Anteroposterior and lateral radiographs of the hip and pelvis are obtained. An intracapsular fracture of the left femoral neck is diagnosed. The patient is admitted for a hemiarthroplasty of the left hip.

## 7.2 Anatomy

The hip joint comprises the head of the femur and the acetabulum of the pelvis (made up of the ischium, ilium and pubis). The capsule of the joint extends to the femoral neck. Anatomical landmarks of the proximal femur include the following (**Figure 7.1**):

- the femoral neck
- the greater trochanter
- the lesser trochanter

The stability of the hip joint is reinforced by ligaments and the acetabular labrum, which deepens the acetabulum, thereby increasing the area in contact with the femoral head. Strong anterior ligaments limit hip extension. The hip capsule is attached to the intertrochanteric line anteriorly and posteriorly 1–2 cm above the intertrochanteric crest (**Figure 7.2**).

### Vascular supply

Most blood supply to the femoral head is provided by the medial and lateral circumflex arteries, which are branches of profunda femoris (**Figure 7.3**). The medial femoral circumflex supplies most of the weight-bearing portion of the femoral

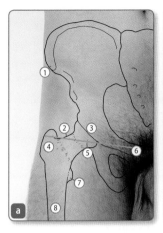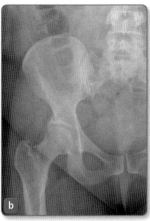

**Figure 7.1** The hip. (a) Surface anatomy. (1) Anterior superior iliac spine, (2) femoral neck, (3) acetabulum overlying femoral head, (4) greater trochanter, (5) midpoint of pubic tubercle-greater trochanter line marking vertical plane of hip joint centre, (6) pubic tubercle-greater trochanter line, (7) lesser trochanter, (8) femoral shaft. (b) Radiograph of the right hip joint.

head. A lesser blood supply is provided by the artery of ligamentum teres. Nutrient vessels from within the femur also contribute to the blood supply.

### Innervation

The femoral, sciatic and gluteal nerves provide sensation around the hip (**Figures 7.4, 7.5** and **7.6**). They may be damaged by trauma or iatrogenically during surgical procedures in this area:

Knowledge of both the motor and sensory functions of these nerves is essential when assessing for neurological deficit (see Table 10.1).

### Surface anatomy

Bony landmarks of the hip and pelvis include the anterior inferior iliac spine, the pubic symphysis and tubercle and the greater trochanter (**Figure 7.1**).

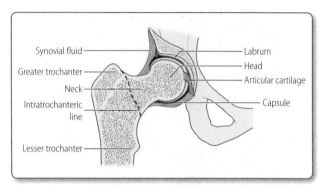

**Figure 7.2** Anatomy of the hip joint.

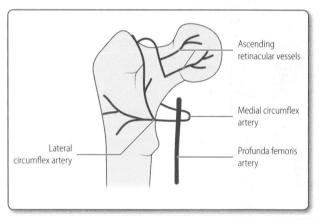

**Figure 7.3** Blood supply to the femoral head.

## 7.3 Examination

### Key signs

Key signs to assess for include pain, reduced range of movement, leg length discrepancies and inability to weight bear.

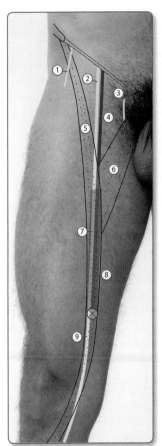

**Figure 7.4** Neurovasculature of the antero-medial right thigh and adductor canal. (1) Lateral cutaneous nerve of the thigh, (2) femoral nerve, (3) obturator nerve, (4) femoral artery, (5) sartorius, (6) adductor longus, (7) saphenous nerve and femoral artery in adductor/subsartorial canal, (8) region of adductor/subsartorial canal (blue), (9) saphenous nerve, ⊗ position of adductor hiatus, ⊗ pubic tubercle.

## Examination sequence

Examination follows a system of 'look, feel and move', along with assessment of function.

### Look

- Look for swelling and bruising around the lateral thigh, groin and gluteal region

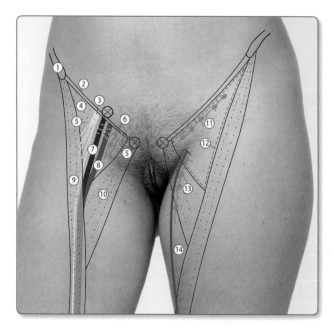

**Figure 7.5** Femoral triangle. ① Anterior superior iliac spine, ② inguinal ligament, ③ femoral nerve, ④ iliopsoas, ⑤ femoral sheath (grey hatch), ⑥ deep inguinal lymph nodes (Cloquet's node in femoral canal), ⑦ femoral artery, ⑧ femoral vein, ⑨ sartorius and subsartorial/adductor canal, ⑩ adductor longus, ⑪ superficial inguinal lymph nodes (proximal group), ⑫ femoral triangle border, ⑬ superficial inguinal lymph nodes (distal group), ⑭ long saphenous vein, Ⓧ midinguinal point, ⊗ pubic tubercle.

- Note any limb shortening
- Note any deformity
- Does the limb appear externally or internally rotated?
- Note the skin colour, and any breaks in the skin

### Feel

- Palpate for bony tenderness over the greater trochanter and the pubic symphysis and tubercle

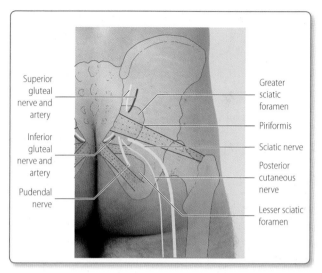

**Figure 7.6** Neurovasculature sites of the hip.

## Move
- Assess active and passive movements
- Can the patient actively carry out a straight leg raise?
- Gently internally and externally rotate the hip
- Extend and flex the hip joint (**Figure 7.7**)
- Abduct and adduct the hip joint

## Function
- Test the nerves for motor and sensory function
- Confirm the dorsalis pedis and posterior tibial pulses
- Can the patient weight-bear?
- Check for pulses along with capillary refill
- Conduct a neurological examination

## 7.4 Hip dislocation

Hip dislocations are most commonly caused by high-energy trauma. The hip dislocates in an anterior or a posterior direction,

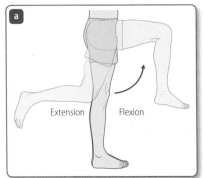

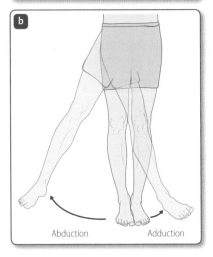

**Figure 7.7** Hip movements: (a) Flexion (115–120°); (b) abduction (45–50°) and adduction (25–30°).

depending on the mechanism. The dislocation is associated with fracture of the femoral head or neck (**Figure 7.8**).

In patients who have undergone hip replacement, the hip may dislocate via a low-energy mechanism. This is often as a consequence of a seemingly trivial manoeuvre, such as bending forwards and twisting on the side on which the hip was replaced.

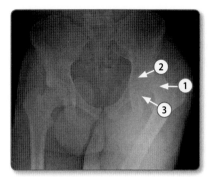

**Figure 7.8** Anteroposterior radiograph of pelvis showing fracture and posterior dislocation of the left hip. The femoral head (1) is not sitting in the acetabulum (2). A small fracture fragment of the femoral head (3) is visible. Compare the appearance of the left hip to that of the normal, right side.

## Epidemiology

Most patients with native hip dislocation have a history of significant trauma. An estimated 50% with hip dislocations also have a fracture.

Posterior dislocations are the most common (80–95% of cases). Sciatic nerve injury is found on presentation in up to 20% of patients with posterior dislocations.

## Causes

The most common causes of hip dislocations are motor vehicle accidents (including dashboard injuries), falls from heights and sports injuries.

Posterior dislocations most frequently result from trauma to a flexed hip and knee. The abducted or externally rotated hip is more likely to dislocate anteriorly.

## Clinical features

Full primary and secondary surveys are required, in accordance with Advanced Trauma Life Support protocol. Concomitant injuries commonly include acetabular, pelvic, femoral head and shaft fractures, as well as patellar, tibial plateau and spinal injuries.

The patient has significant pain in the hip area and is unable to weight-bear. The hip appears shortened.
- A flexed, internally rotated and adducted position implies posterior dislocation

- External rotation with abduction implies an anterior dislocation

Foot drop, if present, indicates sciatic nerve injury. Injury to the femoral nerve and vessels is present only very rarely in cases of anterior dislocation.

The patient is examined for neurological or vascular dysfunction of the lower limb.

## Investigations

Anteroposterior pelvic radiographs are required. A lateral radiograph of the hip is obtained to distinguish an anterior from a posterior dislocation and to assess for pelvic or acetabular fractures. Shenton's lines are usually disrupted if there is also a fracture. Judet views of the acetabulum are also helpful.

A CT scan must be obtained in all cases of traumatic dislocation. This clearly determines the nature of the injury and identifies fractures not visible on radiographs.

Reduction should not be delayed while awaiting the results of further imaging studies, unless these will aid operative planning.

## Management

Urgent reduction, i.e. within 6 h of injury, is required. The risk of avascular necrosis increases with the length of time the hip remains dislocated.

Initially, closed reduction is attempted. Open reduction

### Clinical insight

In contrast to traumatic native hip dislocations, dislocations of total hip replacements and hip hemiarthroplasties are generally caused by low-energy mechanisms. For example, the hip may dislocate when the patient is doing up shoes or turning to get out of a chair or car.

When taking the history, ascertain the contact details of the surgeon who carried out the index procedure; if revision surgery is required knowing the type, make and sizes of implants helps inform surgical planning. Enquire as to the number of previous dislocations, if any, and how the dislocation occurred. Document any neurovascular dysfunction.

Most patients require reduction under general anaesthetic. Closed reduction is usually achieved in theatre under an image intensifier; this enables assessment of the stability of the joint. An orthotic hip brace is usually fitted postoperatively to reduce the likelihood of recurrence.

is required if closed reduction fails. Associated fractures are ideally managed at the same time. Stability is assessed after the reduction.

**Complications** The risk of complications increases with the length of time the hip is dislocated and the complexity of the injury. Common complications include:

- fracture of the femoral head, neck or shaft during reduction
- avascular necrosis of the femoral head
- post-traumatic arthritis
- sciatic nerve injury and resultant palsy
- recurrent dislocation
- infection
- deep vein thrombosis or pulmonary embolism

# 7.5 Neck of femur fractures

Neck of femur fractures (proximal femoral fractures) are the most common fractures encountered by orthopaedic doctors on call. These injuries most commonly occur in elderly people who have had a low-energy fall and are increasingly common.

They are associated with high morbidity and mortality. It has been reported that 10% of patients with a neck of femur fracture die within 1 month, and up to 40% die within 12 months. Generally, even with the best outcome, up to 50% of patients never regain their prefracture level of function.

The high mortality associated with neck of femur fractures reflects the associated comorbidities in the elderly patients affected. The fall and resultant fracture are usually a consequence of many factors, and probably indicate a general decline in health. Most hospitals now have specific guidelines for proximal femoral fractures, and a multidisciplinary team approach to management is emphasised. Patients often spend a long time in hospital as inpatients and require long-term postoperative care.

Neck of femur fractures are classified by anatomical location:

- intracapsular
- extracapsular
- subtrochanteric

### Epidemiology

The incidence of proximal femoral fractures increases with age. Women are affected in 80% of cases. In the younger population, these fractures are rare and more common in men. Hip fractures account for a huge number of orthopaedic admissions. Risk factors for proximal femoral fracture include:

- osteoporosis
- female sex
- advanced age
- multiple comorbidities
- a history of falls
- alcohol use
- malignancy

### Causes

In the elderly population, proximal femoral fractures are almost always the result of a low-energy fall. In younger patients, they are the result of either high-energy trauma associated with polytrauma or stress fractures. Stress fractures of the femoral neck are also encountered in athletes, marathon runners and ballet dancers.

### Clinical features

Patients typically present with:

- pain in the hip, groin or thigh
- inability to weight-bear
- inability to actively carry out a straight leg raise
- bruising
- tenderness around the bony landmarks of the hip
- shortened and externally rotated lower limb
- pain on any attempted movement of the hip

Patients with impacted or stress fractures can have more subtle clinical findings:

- lack of deformity
- pain on weight-bearing
- pain on hip flexion and extension

The patient is assessed for evidence of neurologic or vascular injury.

**Fall history** In elderly patients, a thorough history of the fall is required, as well as past medical history, drug history and social history. This information is used to optimise the patient preoperatively, select the safest anesthetic and for the multidisciplinary team to determine an appropriate care plan following discharge from hospital. The minimum information to ascertain is:

- History or dizziness, chest pain or palpitations
- Any loss of consciousness?
- Does the patient have recurrent falls? If so, has this been investigated?
- What comorbidities exist?
- Have they ever had malignant disease?
- Are they on regular medication? If so, what?
- Are they on anticoagulants? (This treatment may need to be reversed before surgery using local haematology guidelines)
- Where do they live? And who do they live with?
- Are there stairs at home?
- Do they have a carer?
- What are their activities of daily living?
- Do they use a walking aid?

### Investigation

An anteroposterior radiograph of the pelvis and a lateral radiograph of the hip are obtained. Normally, the fracture is obvious. If not, both sides are compared to assess symmetry in Shenton's lines and the angulation of the head to the neck. **Figure 7.9** shows the normal lines, and **Figure 7.10** shows disruption of Shenton's line. If malignancy is possible, full-length radiographs of the femur are required.

If the examination findings are consistent with a fracture but there is no obvious radiographic abnormality, an MRI or CT scan is requested.

Preoperative work-up consists of:
- radiography of the chest
- electrocardiography
- echocardiography

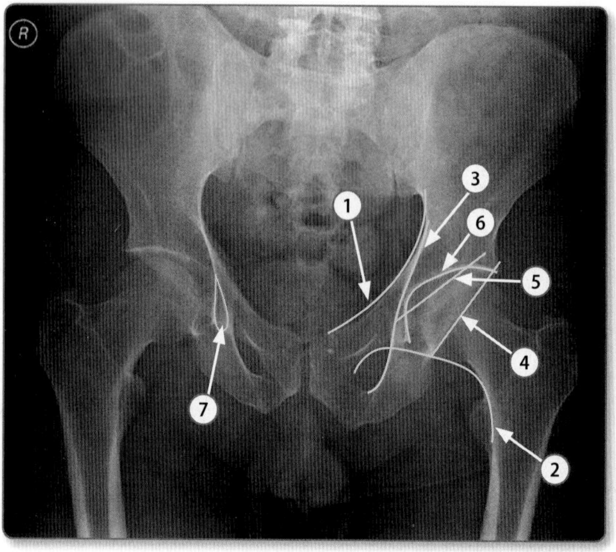

**Figure 7.9** Anteroposterior radiograph of the pelvis, showing normal anatomical lines around the acetabulum. ① Iliopectineal line, ② Shenton's line, ③ ilioischial line, ④ posterior wall acetabulum, ⑤ anterior wall of acetabulum, ⑥ acetabular roof, ⑦ pelvic teardrop.

- full blood count, group and save, urea and electrolytes, international normalised ratio and measurement of blood glucose

## Management

Pain control is paramount, so adequate analgesia should be provided. A 3 in 1 nerve block (femoral, obdurator and lateral cutaneous nerve of thigh) should be considered.

The patient's condition is medically optimised in preparation for surgery. Adequate fluid resuscitation is ensured. If the patient has been lying on the floor for some time after the fall rhabdomyolysis is considered. Renal function must be checked to ensure that it is adequate, and creatine kinase is measured.

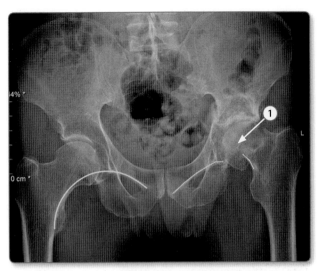

**Figure 7.10** Anteroposterior radiograph of the pelvis showing a displaced subcapital intracapsular fracture of the left femoral neck ①. Shenton's line is disrupted; it is usually a smooth curve (left). Disruption of this line raises the suspicion of fracture.

A plan for definitive surgery is decided as soon as possible, ideally within 36 h. Prompt surgery improves outcomes, relieves pain and minimises the risk of medical complications.

Only patients deemed too unwell to tolerate anaesthesia do not undergo surgery. If there is any doubt, an anaesthetic opinion is sought.

Surgical management of the fracture depends on the nature of the fracture (**Figure 7.11**). The aim of surgery is to stabilise the fracture, thereby reducing pain and restoring function.

### Clinical insight

A multidisciplinary approach, using local guidelines, is used for patients presenting with neck of femur fractures. The aim is to optimise patients preoperatively and rehabilitate them postoperatively, with the aim of them recovering mobility and independence following discharge from hospital.

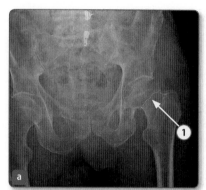

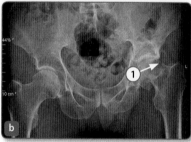

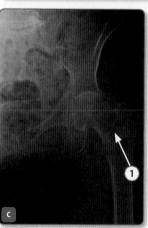

**Figure 7.11** Neck of femur fracturesa. (a) Anteroposterior radiograph of left hip showing a minimally displaced intracapsular fracture of the left femoral neck. (1) Fracture line running across the subcapital region, with minimal displacement of the femoral head. (b) Displaced intracapasular (subcapital) neck of left femur fracture. (1) Fracture line running across subcapital region with displacement of the femoral head. (c) Anteroposterior radiograph of left hip showing an intertrochanteric fracture of the left femoral neck. (1) Fracture line. *Continues oposite.*

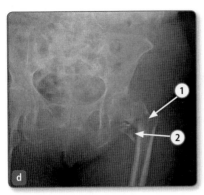

**Figure 7.11** *Continued.* (d) Anteroposterior radiograph of left hip showing a subtrochanteric fracture. ① Complex extracapsular fracture line, ② displaced lesser trochanteric fracture with subtrochanteric extension.

Optimal care of patients with proximal femoral fracture requires multidisciplinary team (MDT) management by:

- an orthopaedic surgeon
- a specialist nurse
- an orthogeriatrician
- a physiotherapist
- a social worker
- occupational therapists

After surgery, the patient's condition is medically optimised; they are then supported to mobilise early. After discharge, intermediate- or long-term care is provided, if appropriate.

**Management of intracapsular fractures** Intracapsular fractures fall into two broad categories:

- displaced
- undisplaced

Their surgical management depends on the degree of displacement (**Figure 7.12**). The most widely used classification is the Garden classification (**Table 7.1** and **Figure 7.13**). Less commonly used is Pauwel's classification (**Table 7.2** and **Figure 7.14**). Intracapsular fractures are described by location (**Figure 7.14**).

The risk of avascular necrosis increases as the fracture displacement increases.

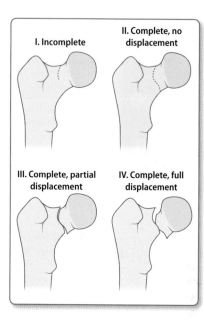

**Figure 7.12** Garden classification of intracapsular fractures.

| Type | I | II | III | IV |
|---|---|---|---|---|
| Degree of valgus displacement and trabecular pattern | Incomplete, non-displaced or valgus impacted Trabeculae angulated | Complete but non-displaced Trabeculae interrupted but not angulated | Complete and marked angulation and disturbance in trabecular pattern | Complete displacement and translation of shaft Complete disruption of trabeculae |

**Table 7.1** Garden classification of intracapsular fractures of the proximal femur.

| Type | I | II | III |
|---|---|---|---|
| Angle fracture forms with horizontal plane (°) | > 30 | 30–70 | > 70 |

**Table 7.2** Pauwel's classification of intracapsular fractures of the proximal femur.

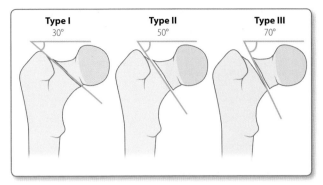

**Figure 7.13** Pauwel's classification of intracapsular fractures.

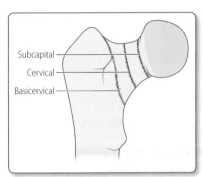

**Figure 7.14** Types of intracapsular fracture.

Subcapital
Cervical
Basicervical

**Management of minimally displaced fractures**  The fracture is reduced, if necessary. Fixation is carried out, usually with three cannulated screws. The principal risk with internal fixation is avascular necrosis.

Generally, postoperative follow-up lasts 2 years, because this is how long avascular necrosis may take to manifest. Radiography is carried out at regular intervals: 6 weeks, 6 months, 12 months, 2 years. Avascular necrosis is usually apparent on radiographs before the onset of symptoms.

The patient is partially weight-bearing for 4–6 weeks after surgery.

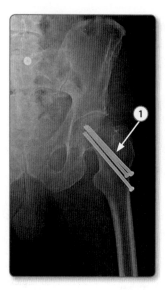

**Figure 7.15** Anteroposterior radiograph of left hip showing a minimally displaced intracapsular fracture of the femoral neck, fixed with three cannulated screws ①.

**Management of displaced fractures** This is a balance between preservation of the native femoral head and the risk of avascular necrosis.

In younger patients, open reduction and internal fixation with cannulated screws or a two-hole dynamic hip screw preserves normal anatomy (**Figure 7.15**). Patients must specifically consent to this procedure, because of the high risk of avascular necrosis. Primary total hip arthroplasty is also considered in the younger population.

In older patients, primary total hip replacement is considered if they:

- can walk independently
- are not cognitively impaired
- are medically fit

If these criteria are not satisfied, cemented hemiarthroplasty is recommended (**Figure 7.16**).

Dislocation is the biggest risk of total hip replacement and hemiarthroplasties. Other risks are infection and injury to the

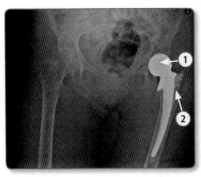

**Figure 7.16** Anteroposterior radiograph of pelvis showing hemiarthroplasty for intracapsular fracture of the femoral neck. ① Thompson's hemiarthroplasty, ② cement surrounding the implant.

sciatic nerve. Full weight-bearing is allowed immediately after total hip arthroplasty or hemiarthroplasty.

**Management of intertrochanteric fractures** By definition, these fractures occur in the anatomical area between the greater and lesser trochanter (see **Figure 7.11c**). This region has a good blood supply, so avascular necrosis is unusual. Intertrochanteric fractures are considered stable or unstable.

For stable fractures:
- dynamic hip screw remains the favoured method of fixation (**Figure 7.17**)
- failure of fixation is a risk of the procedure

For unstable fracture configurations, i.e. reverse oblique:
- an intramedullary nail is more stable (**Figure 7.18**)
- there is a low risk of non-union

**Management of subtrochanteric fractures** These fractures occur between the lesser trochanter and a point 5 cm distal to the lesser trochanter (**Figure 7.19**; see also **Figure 7.11d**). This poorly vascularised region is a common site for pathological fracture.

Subtrochanteric fractures are unstable. There is a high risk of non-union and failure of fixation if they are not recognised and treated appropriately.

These fractures are categorised according to the Fielding classification (**Table 7.3**). An intramedullary device must be

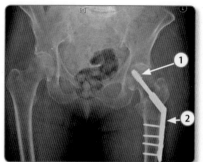

**Figure 7.17**
Anteroposterior radiograph of pelvis showing dynamic hip screw fixation of a left intertrochanteric fracture. ① Compression screw in the femoral head, ② plate with four screws in the proximal femur.

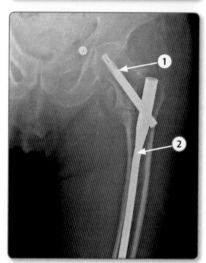

**Figure 7.18**
Anteroposterior radiograph of left hip showing femoral nail fixation of a left subtrochanteric fracture. ① Screw in the femoral head, ② intermedullary nail in the femur.

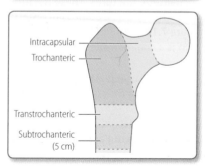

**Figure 7.19** Trochanteric regions of the hip.

Intracapsular
Trochanteric
Transtrochanteric
Subtrochanteric
(5 cm)

| Type | I | II | III |
|---|---|---|---|
| Location of fracture line related to lesser trochanter | At level of lesser trochanter | < 2.5 cm below | 2.5–5 cm below |

**Table 7.3** Fielding classification of subtrochanteric fractures of the proximal femur.

used for their fixation. Specific risks of surgical management of subtrochanteric fractures are non-union, malunion and loss of fixation.

**Complications** More general risks, particularly in elderly patients, are:

- deep vein thrombosis or pulmonary embolism
- wound breakdown
- infection
- decreased mobility compared with the preoperative state
- death

## 7.6 Femoral shaft fractures

The femoral shaft, i.e. the diaphysis, extends from directly beneath the lesser trochanter down to the widening, funnel-shaped section of the distal femur, i.e. the metaphysis.

To aid the description of fracture location, the shaft is often described in terms of thirds: proximal, middle and distal (**Figure 7.20**).

### Epidemiology

The incidence of femoral shaft fractures is bimodal. It peaks in young men and elderly women.

### Causes

In young patients, the mechanism of injury is high-energy trauma, for example from:

- road traffic accidents
- falls from a height

Femoral shaft fractures are often associated with other life-threatening injuries in this patient population.

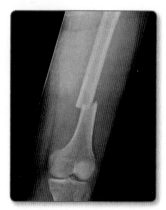

**Figure 7.20** Anteroposterior radiograph of distal femur showing a transverse fracture of the distal femur.

In elderly patients, femoral shaft fractures are usually the result of a fall. Risk factors in this population are:
- osteoporosis
- bony metastases
- use of bisphosphonates

## Clinical features

Patients present with:
- pain in the thigh
- tense swelling
- bruising
- inability to weight-bear
- deformity
- externally rotated and shortened limb
- an open wound (more common in younger patients or secondary to high-energy trauma)

The results of a careful neurovascular examination are documented. A thorough examination of both hip and knee is completed, because ligamentous and meniscal injuries of the ipsilateral knee are present in up to 50% of patients with closed fractures.

## Investigations

Full-length anteroposterior and lateral radiographs of the femur, knee and hip are obtained.

## Management

Management of femoral shaft fractures consists of:
- resuscitation (significant blood loss into the thigh is common)
- transfusion, if required
- taking of blood samples for full blood count and group and save, as soon as possible
- administration of adequate analgesia
- consideration of splinting the fracture

**Conservative management** This is an option only if the patient is unlikely to survive surgery. Conservative management consists of splinting, plaster or traction. Traction is considered in patients awaiting surgery.

**Surgical management** Most patients require operative fixation as soon as possible, ideally within 24 h of presentation.

The surgical options are:
- intramedullary nailing
- plate fixation
- external fixation

Most femoral shaft fractures are treated with intramedullary nailing (**Figure 7.21**).

**Complications** The most common complications are:
- deep vein thrombosis or pulmonary embolism
- infection
- compartment syndrome
- femoral artery or nerve injury
- pudendal nerve injury
- refracture
- non-union or delayed union
- malunion
- knee pain
- heterotopic ossification

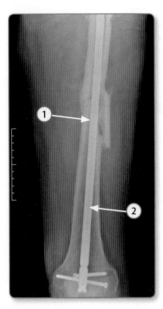

**Figure 7.21** Anteroposterior radiograph of left femur showing a comminuted fracture of the midshaft of the femur ①, treated with insertion of an intermedullary nail ②.

## 7.7 Periprosthetic hip fractures

A periprosthetic fracture is a fracture around an implant. It may occur intraoperatively or at any time afterwards. Loosening around the prosthesis and poor-quality bone increase the risk of periprosthetic fracture.

These fractures tend to occur in the elderly and are a challenge to manage operatively. They are broadly categorised according to the Vancouver classification (**Figure 7.22**):

- type A (trochanteric)
- type B (around the stem)
- type C (entirely distal to the stem)

### Epidemiology

The incidence is higher in elderly patients because they have already required arthroplasty.

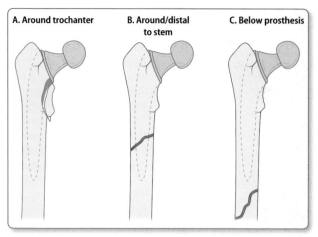

| A. Around trochanter | B. Around/distal to stem | C. Below prosthesis |

**Figure 7.22** Vancouver classification of periprosthetic hip fractures.

The femur is the most frequent site of periprosthetic fracture. The fracture occurs around a hip or knee replacement – sometimes both. The frequency of such fractures is increasing with the number of hip and knee implants. The reported incidence is 1.1% after primary hip replacement.

### Causes
Periprosthetic hip fractures are a consequence of differences in the properties of bone and prosthesis. When force is applied, areas of highly concentrated stress ('stress risers') develop at a point in the bone at the junction between the tip of the rigid, inelastic prosthesis and the elastic bone.

When sufficient force is applied, a fracture occurs at the stress risers. Because stress is highly concentrated at these areas, little energy is required to create a fracture. Osteoporosis, osteolysis and other causes of bone loss around the implant may enable a fracture to occur with minimal energy.

## Clinical insight

The diagnosis of osteoarthritis is usually obvious because of the chronicity of the symptoms and gradual deterioration of the joint. However, other diagnoses to consider are:

**t**rauma

**s**eptic arthritis

**c**rystal arthropathy

**r**heumatoid arthritis

**r**eactive arthritis

### Clinical features

Patients with a periprosthetic fracture present with pain. They are usually unable to weight-bear. There is a history of previous surgery for implantation of the prosthesis. An operative scar is present. The hip may have been painful before the fracture, indicating that the prosthesis was loose.

### Investigations

Anteroposterior and lateral radiographs of the hip and full-length radiographs of the femur are obtained. Due to artefact from the prosthesis, CT and MRI scans are difficult to interpret.

During surgery, tissue samples are taken for biopsy if infection or a pathological cause of fracture is suspected.

### Management

The fracture is managed surgically, either by fixation or revision arthroplasty surgery. The decision to fix a fracture or revise the prosthesis depends on the site, nature and extent of the fracture, and whether the prosthesis is fixed or loose. Some periprosthetic fractures occur in the presence of infection.

## 7.8 Osteoarthritis

Osteoarthritis is a chronic disease of the joints; it is characterised by degeneration of cartilage and bone, and causes pain and stiffness. It usually, but not exclusively, affects weight-bearing joints.

### Epidemiology

Osteoarthritis is the most common joint disease. Risk factors include:

- advanced age
- family history of osteoarthritis
- obesity
- female sex

## Causes

The cause of primary osteoarthritis is unknown, but it is thought to be associated with 'overworking' the affected joint. In some cases, there is a genetic component.

Secondary osteoarthritis affects younger people and typically follows:

- Perthes' disease (Legg–Calvé–Perthes disease)
- slipped upper femoral epiphysis
- avascular necrosis
- developmental dislocation of the hip
- traumatic dislocation of the hip
- infection

See Chapter 9 for a description of the features of osteoarthritis (page 265).

## Clinical features

Patients present with pain localised around the groin, hip, trochanter or buttocks. The pain is occasionally referred to the knee or back. The hip is often stiff, with functional impairment; the patient may struggle to cut their toenails or put on their shoes and socks. There is reduced range of motion at the hip. Sleep disturbance secondary to pain is common.

## Investigations

An anteroposterior pelvic radiograph for both hips is obtained, as well as a lateral radiograph of the symptomatic hip. The classic findings are those described in Chapter 9 (page 265; **Figure 7.23**). Radiographic findings may not correlate with the level of symptoms.

## Management

Osteoarthritis is initially, and sometimes definitively, managed conservatively. Surgical management is with joint arthoplasty.

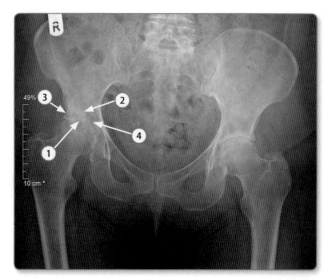

**Figure 7.23** Anteroposterior radiograph of pelvis showing osteoarthritis of the left hip. ① Loss of superior joint space, ② subchondral sclerosis (the increased density manifests as whiteness adjacent to the joint surfaces), osteophyte ③, cyst formation ④.

**Conservative management** Initial management consists of analgesia, weight loss (if appropriate), modification of activity (reduction in impact activities, walking aids) and physical therapy.

**Surgical management** Arthritis of the hip is managed by joint replacement surgery (arthroplasty). Because of the good longevity of hip implants, surgery is generally considered at an earlier stage than in previous years. Surgery has the potential to significantly improve patients' quality of life.

**Complications** The complications of osteoarthritis of the hip are:

· dislocation
· loosening

- osteolysis
- nerve and blood vessel injury
- shortened leg, resulting in length discrepancy

---

## 7.9 Paget's disease of bone

Paget's disease of bone (originally termed osteitis deformans) is a disorder of bone remodelling. Accelerated bone turnover results in a disorganised bone matrix; it is coarse, with increased vascularity. The affected bone is more prone to fracture.

The process is usually localised to a single bone. The affected bone becomes deformed in consequence.

### Epidemiology

The disease is most common in northern Europe. It is nearly twice as common in men than women, and usually develops in the patient's forties.

### Causes

There may be a genetic component to the condition. Slow virus infection (paromyxovirus) has been implicated as a cause.

### Clinical features

Paget's disease of bone generally remains asymptomatic for many years. Patients usually complain of pain, which is often misdiagnosed as arthritic pain from the hip. Deep bone pain is what the patients describe.

The condition is typically diagnosed incidentally when a radiograph of the hip is obtained for other reasons. It may present with a pathological fracture. The skin over the affected area may feel warm.

### Investigations

Plain radiography shows the characteristic features of Paget's disease of bone:
- lytic lesions and sclerosis, concurrently or separately
- coarse trabeculae
- thickened cortex

A bone scan accurately marks the site of disease and shows increased activity in affected bone. Blood tests show an increased level of alkaline phosphatase.

### Management

Simple analgesia is required for the symptomatic patient. If the patient has presented with a pathological fracture, this is fixed. If surgery is planned, there is a higher risk of bleeding because of the increased vascularity of the bone.

Management of the disease in its early stages, before there is significant bone deformity, is associated with an improved prognosis.

Total hip replacement is the most common procedure in the presence of Paget's disease of bone and arthritis. This procedure carries a higher risk of complications because of the increased risk of bleeding and the deformity of the femur that is often present.

Paget's sarcoma is a rare bone tumour that occurs in about 5% of all patients with long-standing polyostotic disease.

## 7.10 Other conditions

### Femoral head fractures

Nearly all fractures of the femoral head are associated with hip dislocations and occur as a result of high-energy trauma. The injury is visible on anteroposterior pelvic and lateral hip radiographs. CT imaging yields further information.

The Pipkin classification is most commonly used to categorise this type of fracture. The most serious and common complication is avascular necrosis; for some patients, the risk is up to 50%. **Figure 7.7** shows a Pipkin type I fracture dislocation of the hip.

### Prosthetic joint infection

Prosthetic joint infection is a serious condition. Ideally, it is treated by surgeons who manage revision arthroplasty on a regular basis.

Management of infected joint replacements requires a multidisciplinary approach. As part of initial management, radiographs of the hip are obtained:

- anteroposterior pelvis for both hips
- lateral hip
- full-length femur

Blood cultures and blood samples (including full blood count, urea and electrolytes, C-reactive protein, erythrocyte sedimentation rate) are required. Antibiotics are not started unless at the specific instruction of senior colleagues. If aspiration of the hip is considered, this is also carried out in a clean air environment.

# Pelvis

The pelvis is the lower part of the trunk, where the axial skeleton connects to the lower limbs. The bony pelvis is a ring formed by the two innominate (or hip) bones, joined by the sacrum posteriorly and the pubic symphysis anteriorly. It transfers load to the lower limbs by way of the articulation with both femora, provides muscular attachments, and contains and protects the lower abdominal and pelvic viscera.

Multiple vessels traverse the pelvis. Haemorrhage from an unstable pelvic injury may be from bone, arteries or veins.

## 8.1 Clinical scenario

### A fall from a horse

#### Background

A 59-year-old woman has sustained injuries from a fall from a horse and the horse subsequently falling on to her while she lay on the ground. She complains of lower abdominal and pelvic pain, particularly on movement, and says she feels nauseated and light-headed.

#### Examination

On primary survey, the patient's condition is unstable; she has low blood pressure and persistent tachycardia. These improve with application of a pelvic binder. She has pain on palpation of the pelvis. Sensation is normal in all four limbs, and all peripheral pulses are present.

After being given a unit of red blood cells, her blood pressure stabilises. She is transferred to the nearest emergency department.

She has no past medical history of note.

#### Differential diagnosis

The possible injuries are:

- pelvic fracture with or without vascular injury
- abdominal or chest injury
- long bone fracture

Given the mechanism of injury, hypotension and acute pain, a pelvic injury is most likely.

### Investigations

Imaging studies are carried out on arrival at the emergency department. They include radiography of the chest and pelvis, confirming a pelvic fracture. She undergoes a CT with contrast that shows a bleed from a branch of the internal iliac artery: it is embolised by the radiologist.

The binder remains in situ while the patient undergoes a full examination. Her condition is stabilised before she is sent to theatre for application of a pelvic external fixator.

## 8.2 Anatomy

The pelvis is a strong, stable bony structure that connects the trunk to the lower limbs. Its functions are to protect the pelvic contents and to transmit the weight of the upper body and spine to the lower limbs.

The pelvis comprises the sacrum, coccyx, and the ischium, ilium and pubic bone of each hip bone (**Figure 8.1, 8.2** and **8.3**). The acetabulum is a concave cup formed by the ilium, the ischium and the pubic bone and articulates with the femoral head to form the hip joint.

The main joints of the pelvis itself are the symphysis pubis and the two sacroiliac joints. When viewed either inferiorly or superiorly, the bones of the intact pelvis form a complete ovoid ring.

### Vascular supply and innervation

The pelvis has a complex neurovascular supply. Its main source of innervation is the lumbosacral plexus, and its main source of blood is the internal iliac artery.

### Surface anatomy

The pelvis has many bony landmarks.

- Anteriorly, it is possible to palpate the anterior superior iliac spine, the iliac crest, the pubic tubercle and the symphysis pubis (**Figure 8.1**)

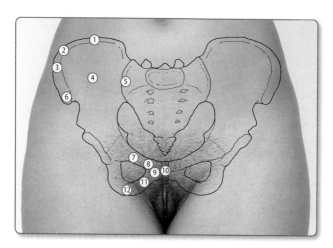

**Figure 8.1** Bones of the anterior female pelvis. (1) Highest point of iliac crest (supracristal plane), (2) iliac crest, (3) tubercle of iliac crest, (4) iliac bone, (5) sacroiliac joint, (6) anterior superior iliac spine, (7) superior pubic ramus, (8) pubic tubercle, (9) body of pubis, (10) pubic symphysis, (11) inferior pubic ramus, (12) ischial tuberosity.

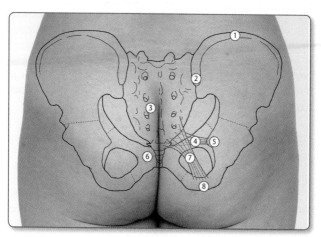

**Figure 8.2** Bones and ligaments of the posterior female pelvis. (1) Highest point of iliac crest (supracristal plane), (2) posterior superior iliac spine, (3) sacrum, (4) sacrospinous ligament, (5) ischial spine, (6) coccyx, (7) sacrotuberous ligament, (8) ischial tuberosity.

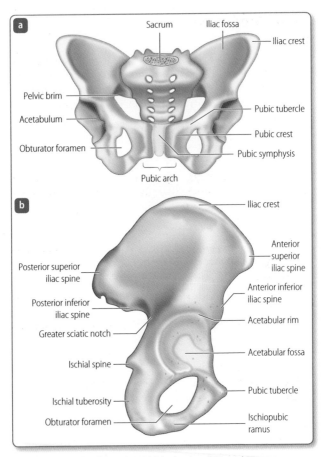

**Figure 8.3** Anatomy of the pelvis. (a) Anterior view. (b) Lateral view.

- Posteriorly, the posterior superior iliac spine, iliac crests, sacroiliac joints, ischial tuberosities and lumbosacral spine can be palpated (**Figure 8.2**)

## 8.3 Examination

### Key signs

Key signs to assess for include pain, and movement of the hips and lower limbs. Gentle anteroposterior and lateral compression of the pelvis will elicit the pain. Blood at the external urethral meatus is a sign of a pelvic fracture in trauma patients unless proved otherwise. Always look for signs of shock in trauma patients.

### Examination sequence

Examination follows a system of 'Look, feel and move', and test of function. Imaging studies are required if injury is suspected, as the pelvis cannot be fully examined externally.

### Look

- Are there any obvious bruises, abrasions or wounds over the pelvis?
- Is there any leg length discrepancy?
- Are the legs well perfused, warm and with a capillary return of less than 2 s to the toes?
- Is there any bleeding or bruising at the external genitalia?

### Feel

- Palpate the pelvis for pain
- Feel to assess distal pulses and skin warmth
- Check for sensation of the lower limbs

### Move

- Look for pain on axial loading or movement of the hips
- Compress the pelvis gently in both the coronal and sagittal planes

### Function:

- Is the patient able to weight bear?

## 8.4 Pelvic fractures

A pelvic fracture is classed as 'unstable' if the pelvic ring is broken in two or more places; in contrast, an isolated fracture is classed as 'stable'. Pelvic fractures are generally considered unstable, because it is unusual for a fracture to be present in one part of the ring without disruption to another. The second injury may not always be bony; it may be ligamentous and possibly occult.

### Epidemiology

Pelvic fractures are most commonly sustained by young men (aged 15–28 years) and elderly women (aged > 75 years).

### Causes

The complete pattern of injury is sought. In younger patients, pelvic fractures are usually caused by high-energy trauma, for example from road traffic accidents, falls from heights or crush injuries. Such injuries are unstable and associated with high mortality as a consequence of haemorrhage and associated injuries.

In the elderly population, pelvic fractures are usually caused by low-energy falls and are therefore more stable than such fractures in younger people. Young athletes may have stable fractures as a result of avulsion. Avulsion fractures are chronic injuries caused by repeated vigorous muscle contraction. For example, footballers may sustain fracture of the anterior inferior iliac spine from avulsion of the rectus femoris, or fracture of the ischium from avulsion of the hamstrings.

### Clinical features

Seventy-five per cent of patients with unstable pelvic fractures are also haemodynamically unstable and in a poor physiological condition. Other life-threatening injuries to the head, spine, chest and abdomen, and long-bone fractures are common. Therefore they require full initial assessment in accordance with the Advanced Trauma Life Support (ATLS) approach or a similar protocol.

Bruising over the flank or buttocks indicates a significant haemorrhage. Patients occasionally have leg length discrepancy or rotational deformity. There is usually tenderness on palpation of the pelvis anteriorly, posteriorly or laterally.

If pelvic injury is suspected, the perineum must be examined to check for an open fracture and for rectal, vaginal or urethral injury. A full neurological examination of the lower limbs is carried out to exclude injury to the lumbosacral plexus.

If pelvic injury was suspected at the scene of an accident or in the emergency department, a pelvic binder will have been applied or required as part of initial haemorrhage control. The presence of a pelvic binder can make examination of a patient more difficult.

### Investigations

Pelvic injuries are associated with significant haemorrhage, so haemodynamic status is assessed and the patient resuscitated before further examination. If they remain haemodynamically unstable, immediate surgical exploration or interventional radiology (CT angiography and embolisation) are necessary before further examination or investigation.

An anteroposterior radiograph of the pelvis is usually requested as part of an initial trauma series. For pelvic ring fractures, pelvic inlet and outlet views are useful to determine anterior or posterior displacement and vertical displacement, respectively. CT scans are useful to assess pelvic injuries. If the patient's condition is stable, MRI has a role, particularly in assessing for genitourinary and vascular injuries.

### Management

Before the initiation of specific pelvic management, the patient needs to be resuscitated

## Clinical insight

In cases of suspected pelvic ring injury, a systematic assessment of pelvic radiographs is required (**Figure 8.8**).

1. Look closely at the pelvic ring
2. Assess the obturator foramina
3. Compare the widths of the sacroiliac joints; they should be equal
4. Assess the symphysis pubis; it should be < 5 mm, and there should be no widening
5. Inspect the arcuate lines of the sacral foramina and compare sides
6. Look at the acetabulum in detail

A fracture at one site is likely to be associated with disruption at another site.

## Clinical insight

Six lines are assessed when reviewing a pelvic radiograph:

- The iliopectineal line, to evaluate the anterior column
- The ilioischial line, to evaluate the posterior column
- The dome of the acetabulum
- The 'teardrop', to evaluate the anteroinferior portion of the acetabular fossa
- The anterior rim of the acetabulum
- The posterior rim of the acetabulum

in accordance with the ATLS protocol. It must be ensured that blood samples have been obtained for group and save and crossmatching. If an unstable pelvic ring injury is suspected, a pelvic binder is applied.

Senior colleagues are placed in charge of the patient's care: each case requires discussion with a major trauma centre and usually require an urgent transfer there once the patient is stable. Even fractures that appear minor can be associated with life-threatening injuries. In cases of ongoing arterial haemorrhage, CT angiography and embolisation are required before further management.

The Young–Burgess classification is the most widely used system for categorising pelvic fractures; it is based on the mechanism of injury and forces applied (**Table 8.1**). The three main types of fracture pattern described are anterior posterior compression (APC) (**Figure 8.4**), lateral compression (LC) (**Figure 8.5**) and vertical shear (VS) (**Figure 8.6**). Categorisation of the degree of injury is used to guide conservative or surgical management and helps prevent missed lesions.

The open book pelvic injury, from an anterior posterior compression injury, is a rotationally unstable and vertically stable pattern.

### Conservative management

Isolated fractures of the pubic rami, APC I and LC I fractures (in which the anterior gap is < 2.5 cm and posterior injury is minimal) are all stable fractures and only minimally displaced. They are managed by bed rest, with weight-bearing allowed, with crutches initially, as pain tolerates. Regular radiographs are obtained to ensure that there is no displacement of the fracture.

| Type | Description | Treatment |
|------|-------------|-----------|
| APC I | Symphysis widening < 2.5 cm or anterior vertical fracture pattern of rami; all sacroiliac ligaments intact | Non-operative: protected weight-bearing |
| APC II | Symphysis widening > 2.5 cm, anterior sacroiliac joint (sacrotuberous and sacrospinous ligaments) diastasis; posterior sacroiliac ligaments intact | Anterior symphyseal plate or external fixator |
| APC III | Disruption of whole anterior and posterior sacroiliac ligaments (sacroiliac dislocation), often associated with vascular and nerve injury | Anterior symphyseal plate or external fixator and posterior stabilisation |
| LC I | Minor anterior fracture with small sacral ala compression fracture | Non-operative: protected weight-bearing |
| LC II | Rami fracture and ipsilateral posterior crescent-shaped fracture of iliac wing at or near anterior border of sacroiliac joint | Open reduction and internal fixation of ilium |
| LC III | Ipsilateral LC and contralateral APC: complete posterior injury, normally as a result of initial impact and secondary crush | Posterior stabilisation with plate or screws |
| VS | Posterior and superior directed force; vertical displacement of hemipelvis; associated with highest risk of haemorrhage and death | Posterior stabilisation with plate or screws |
| CM | When factors not readily apparent: any combination of the above injuries; patterns vary | Depends on fracture pattern combinations |

APC, anterior posterior compression; CM, combined mechanical; LC, lateral compression; VS, vertical shear.

**Table 8.1** Young–Burgess classification of pelvic fractures.

**Surgical management** For pelvic ring fractures in which the anterior gap is > 2.5 cm, surgical management is required. External fixators are used for APC and VS fractures, and also as part of haemorrhage control in emergency situations.

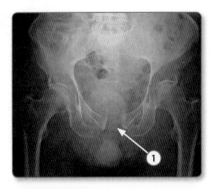

**Figure 8.4**
Anteroposterior pelvic radiograph showing a pelvic fracture caused by anterior posterior compression (1).

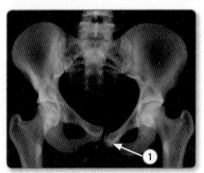

**Figure 8.5**
Anteroposterior pelvic radiograph showing a pelvic fracture caused by lateral compression. Disruption of the pelvic ring (1) is particularly evident at the symphysis pubis, indicating lateral compression.

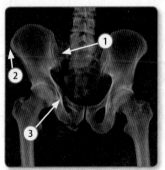

**Figure 8.6** Anteroposterior pelvic radiograph showing a vertical shear pelvic fracture: fracture through the rami and sacrum, with cephalad displacement. (1) Sacral fracture, (2) cephalad displacement of right hemipelvis, (3) fracture through the rami.

Definitive treatment is almost always required. Surgical options include open reduction and internal fixation, either acute or delayed, with combinations of screws and plates (**Figure 8.8**). Some fractures are amenable to less invasive approaches for reduction and fixation.

Other surgical teams may be needed if any other pelvic injuries are suspected. They may include urologists, general surgeons and vascular surgeons.

> ### Clinical insight
>
> Pubic rami fractures (**Figure 8.7**) are very common in the elderly; they are sought in pelvic radiographs of patients who have had a fall, are complaining of hip pain or have difficulty weight-bearing but no evidence of fracture of the neck or femur. Treatment is rest, analgesia and weight-bearing as pain tolerates. These injuries are stable low-energy injuries. Patients are usually admitted for rehabilitation under the care of the medical team, because no orthopaedic input is required.

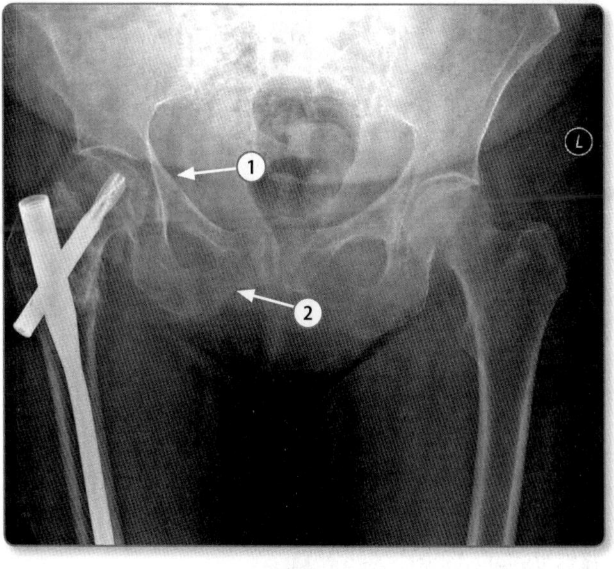

**Figure 8.7** Anteroposterior pelvic radiograph showing a superior and inferior pubic ramus fracture (with previous proximal femoral nailing). ① Fracture of the superior pubic ramus, ② fracture of the inferior pubic ramus.

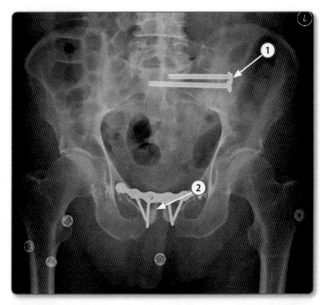

**Figure 8.8** Anteroposterior pelvic radiograph showing open reduction and internal fixation of an open book pelvis. ① Reduction and fixation of the sacroiliac joint. ② Reduction and fixation of the symphysis pubis.

**Complications** Common complications of pelvic fractures are:

- retroperitoneal haemorrhage
- neurological injuries as a result of lumbosacral plexus injuries
- bladder injuries
- urethral injuries
- bowel injuries
- deep vein thrombosis and pulmonary embolism
- chronic instability
- malunion or non-union
- death

## 8.5 Acetabular fractures

Acetabular fractures usually occur as a consequence of high-energy trauma in young patients (e.g. fall from a height or road traffic accident), when the head of the femur is forced into the socket of the hip joint. Acetabular fractures require careful evaluation and precise management; being inta-articular the prevention of degenerative joint disease is paramount. In older patients, acetabular fractures occur with lower energy involved.

## Epidemiology
Acetabular fractures are rare but serious injuries. They are strongly associated with nerve injuries.

## Causes
Fractures of the acetabulum occur after a direct blow to the hip socket through the trochanter, or indirectly through the knee or foot.

## Clinical features
Patients are assessed in accordance with the ATLS protocol. Patients with acetabular fractures have hip or groin pain and are unable to mobilise. Patients may also have associated urological or nerve injuries.

> ### Clinical insight
> Hip dislocation associated with acetabular fracture is an orthopaedic emergency and occurs in up to 30% of acetabular fractures. The hip needs to be relocated urgently (see Chapter 7.4).

## Investigations
An anteroposterior view and two Judet views (iliac oblique and obturator oblique) are required. **Figure 8.9** shows key landmarks to assess on the anteroposterior radiograph. The Iliac view is used to assess the posterior column and the anterior wall (**Figure 8.10**). The obturator view is best for evaluating the anterior column and posterior wall (**Figure 8.11**).

Acetabular fractures are usually comminuted. **Figure 8.12** shows a left acetabular fracture. To further assess the fracture and to improve understanding of the fracture patterns, a CT is requested, including three-dimensional reconstructions, if possible. A CT scan is the investigation of choice for delineating the fracture pattern precisely and for surgical planning.

## Management
The Judet–Letournel classification is used most commonly to describe the ten basic fracture patterns (five elemental and five

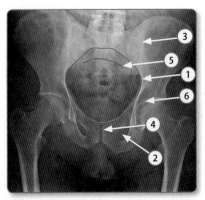

**Figure 8.9**
Anteroposterior pelvic radiograph showing features to identify when reviewing a pelvic anteroposterior radiograph. (1) Pelvic ring, (2) obdurator foramen, (3) sacroiliac joints, (4) symphysis pubis, (5) sacral arcuate lines, (6) acetabulum.

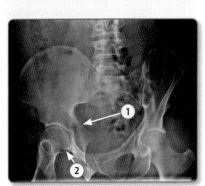

**Figure 8.10** Iliac oblique Judet view radiograph. (1) Ilioschial line (posterior) column, (2) anterior wall of the acetabulum.

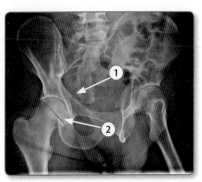

**Figure 8.11** Obdurator oblique Judet view radiograph. (1) Iliopectineal line (anterior column), (2) posterior wall of the acetabulum.

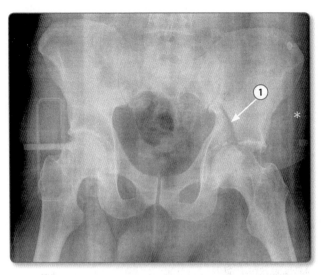

**Figure 8.12** Anteroposterior radiograph showing a left acetabular fracture ①.

associated) defined by the three standard radiographic films.
Elemental patterns:
- posterior wall
- posterior column
- anterior wall
- anterior column
- transverse

Associated patterns:
- associated both column
- transverse plus posterior wall
- T-shaped
- anterior column or wall plus posterior hemitransverse
- posterior column plus posterior wall

This fracture classification enables accurate interpretation of radiographs to help determine the appropriate surgical approach and treatment.

Acetabular fractures are initially managed with analgesia and placement in either skin or skeletal traction. The aims are to facilitate bony union and early movement, and more importantly, to restore the congruency of the hip joint and thereby prevent post-traumatic arthritis.

**Conservative management**  This is appropriate if:

- there is minimal displacement (< 2 mm)
- the femoral head remains congruent in the acetabulum
- the roof arcs of the fractures are > 45°
- the posterior wall fractures cover < 20%

The patient is allowed to toe-touch weight-bear for 6–8 weeks, and regular radiographs are obtained to check that no displacement has occurred. Touch-toe weight bearing allows the toes to be placed on the ground for balance but should not support any weight.

**Surgical management**  This is used for fractures with > 2 mm displacement or loss of joint congruency, posterior wall fractures with fragments > 20%, and fractures with any intra-articular loose bodies or associated fracture dislocations. Early operative treatment has the best outcomes. However, if the patient is stable, it is a closed injury and there are no neurological deficits, surgery can be delayed for up to 2 weeks. The patient remains in traction until surgery. Surgery may be carried out percutaneously with column screws. If open surgery is done, a single surgical approach is preferred.

**Complications**  Common complications of acetabular fractures are:

- injury of the sciatic, femoral and superior gluteal nerve
- avascular necrosis
- post-traumatic arthritis
- heterotopic ossification
- deep vein thrombosis and pulmonary embolism

## 8.6 Sacral fractures

Sacral fractures are easily missed; they therefore often go undiagnosed and mistreated. Twenty-five per cent of sacral fractures have an associated neurological deficit. They are also often associated with injuries to the pelvic ring.

## Causes

As with pelvic fractures, young patients sustain sacral fractures as a result of high-energy trauma, most commonly falls from heights. Sacral fractures in elderly patients are usually the result of low-energy falls.

## Clinical features

Patients present with:
- generalised pelvic pain
- inability to weight bear, or difficulty weight bearing
- neurological deficit

A full trauma survey is completed if the fracture is the result of high-energy trauma. In addition, the findings of a careful neurovascular examination are documented, because > 25% of sacral fractures have an associated nerve injury, and these are frequently missed (S1–S4 pass through the sacral foramina). The perineum of patients with a sacral fracture is also examined.

## Investigations

Anteroposterior pelvic radiographs and inlet and outlet radiographs are obtained. Inlet views are taken anteroposteriorly with a 25° caudal tilt; they are used to analyse the pubic symphysis and pelvic rim. Outlet views enable evaluation of any vertical shift and are taken anteroposteriorly with the beam tilted 35° distally. The arcuate lines that form the margins of the sacral foramina are assessed (**Figure 8.10**); this includes comparison of both sides. Sacral fractures may not be visible on radiographs, so CT is used (or MRI if there is concern about neurological symptoms) (**Figure 8.13**).

## Management

The fractures are transverse or involve the sacral ala. Transverse fractures are more likely to be associated with nerve injury.

**Conservative management**  Most sacral fractures are treated non-operatively, with bed rest and progressive weight-bearing.

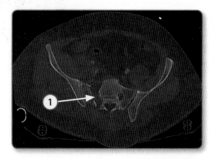

**Figure 8.13** Axial CT scan showing a fracture through the sacral ala ①.

**Surgical management**  For displaced fractures > 1 cm, open injuries or persistent pain and any neurological injury, surgical fixation with decompression is required.

**Complications**  The complications of sacral injuries are:
- deep vein thrombosis or pulmonary embolism
- nerve injury
- malreduction

## 8.7 Coccygeal fractures

This type of fracture most commonly results from a fall on to the buttocks. The injury can be very painful or tender, especially when the patient tries to sit down. The coccyx appears abnormal and angulated on radiographs.

The mainstay of treatment is analgesia, helping the patient to be comfortable and avoidance of constipation with regular laxatives and a high-fibre diet. The patient may find it helpful to sit on rubber ring. If the pain fails to improve, the area is injected with local anaesthetic, or as a last resort, the coccyx can be excised.

# Knee

The knee is one of the largest joints in the body. It is a modified hinge synovial joint; it can flex and extend, and also allows a small degree of internal and external rotation. It supports nearly all the weight of the body, and is therefore at risk of both acute injury and degeneration.

The most common knee injuries are :

- soft tissue injuries, e.g. ACL rupture, normally sustained when playing sport
- patella dislocations, which can be low energy injuries but are often recurrent due to the patient's anatomy
- tibial plateau fractures, which are associated with high energy trauma

Degenerative diseases include osteoarthritis which causes progressive pain, stiffness, swelling and reduced mobility and has a high incidence of up to 240 per 100,000 person years.

## 9.1 Clinical scenario

### Knee injury

#### Background

A 28-year-old man was playing football. He was running with the ball and turned suddenly. His knee buckled and he sustained a twisting injury to the knee, which resulted in immediate swelling. After being assisted off the pitch he went home and over the next 2 weeks the swelling appeared to reduce. He is still, however, experiencing ongoing pain and occasionally feels the knee 'give way'. He decides to visit his local emergency department.

#### History

He is otherwise fit and well. He takes no regular medication. He works as a solicitor, lives with his partner and plays football twice a week.

## Examination

On examination there is no obvious deformity. He has an effusion (also known as water on the knee). His range of movement is 0° to 120° (compared with -5° to 135° on the contra-lateral knee). He has no joint line tenderness. The Lachman test is positive as is the anterior draw test. He has no opening on stressing the medial or lateral collateral ligaments.

## Differential diagnosis

Possible injuries are:

- ACL rupture
- Meniscal tear
- PCL injury
- Osteoarthritis

The most likely diagnosis is ACL rupture, which is often secondary to a twisting/pivot injury and leads to immediate swelling. With meniscal tears patients usually develop swelling overnight. Ongoing instability also indicates a ligament injury.

## Investigations

Anteroposterior and lateral radiographs of the knee are requested to rule out any fracture or arthritic changes. An MRI scan is also arranged. The patient is prescribed analgesia and referred to physiotherapy while waiting on results from the MRI scan and confirmation of diagnosis.

# 9.2 Anatomy

The knee joint compromises four bones: the femur, patella, tibia and fibula (**Figure 9.1, 9.2** and **9.3**) . These are joined at three articulations: the patellofemoral, the tibiofemoral and the tibiofibular. The patella is a sesamoid bone, because of this it is the last of the knee bones to ossify.

The stability of the knee joint is maintained by the ligaments, muscles and tendons and the synovial joint capsule. The knee has two fibrocartilage menisci, the semilunar cartilages, which encircle the medial and lateral tibial condyles; they protect the bony surfaces, increase stability and act as shock absorbers.

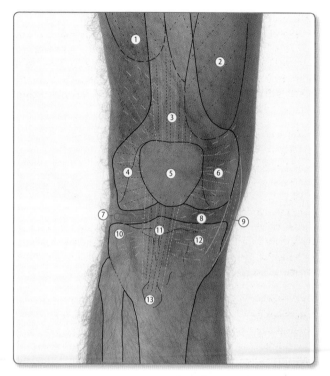

**Figure 9.1** Anterior view of the right knee. ① Vastus lateralis, ② vastus medialis, ③ quadriceps tendon, ④ lateral femoral condyle, ⑤ patella, ⑥ medial femoral condyle, ⑦ lateral meniscus, ⑧ medial meniscus, ⑨ medial (tibial) collateral ligament, ⑩ lateral tibial condyle, ⑪ patellar ligament, ⑫ medial tibial condyle, ⑬ tibial tuberosity.

Numerous bursae surround the knee, the largest of which is the suprapatellar bursa.

## Patella

The patella runs in the patellofemoral groove (trochlea). The quadriceps tendon inserts into the superior pole, and the patellar tendon originates in the inferior pole and runs down to its

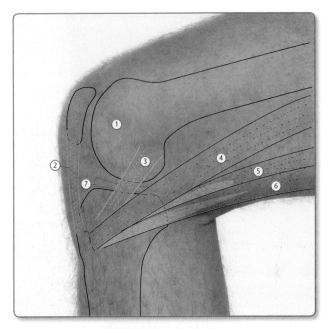

**Figure 9.2** Medial view of the right knee. ① Medial femoral condyle, ② patellar ligament, ③ medial (tibial) collateral ligament, ④ sartorius, ⑤ gracilis and tendon, ⑥ semitendinosus and tendon, ⑦ medial meniscus.

insertion in the tibial tubercle. The patella protects the articular surface of the knee and offers a mechanical advantage to the quadriceps tendon.

## Quadriceps

The quadriceps muscle group comprises rectus femoris, vastus medialis, vastus lateralis and vastus intermedius. These join at the superior patellar border and act in continuity with the patella and patellar ligament to form the extensor mechanism of the lower leg (**Figure 9.4**).

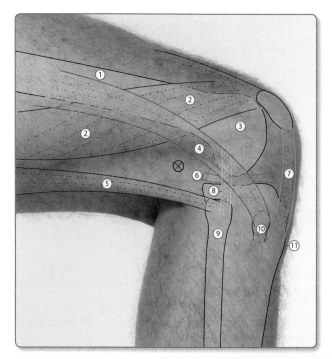

**Figure 9.3** Lateral view of the right knee. ① Femoral shaft, ② vastus lateralis, ③ lateral femoral condyle, ④ iliotibial tract/band, ⑤ biceps femoris, ⑥ lateral meniscus, ⑦ patellar ligament, ⑧ lateral (fibular) collateral ligament, ⑨ fibular head and neck, ⑩ Gerdy's tubercle, ⑪ tibial tuberosity, ⊗ needle insertion point for tibial and common fibular nerve block.

## Ligaments

The knee is stabilised by four ligaments: the anterior and posterior cruciate ligaments, and the medial and collateral ligaments (**Figure 9.5**). The medial and lateral meniscus increases joint congruency and acts as a shock absorber between the tibial plateau and the distal femur.

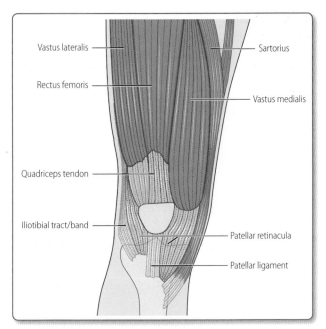

**Figure 9.4** Muscles of the quadriceps.

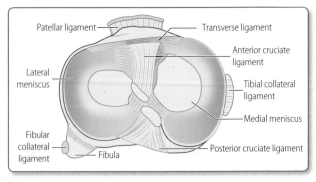

**Figure 9.5** Anatomy of ligaments of the knee.

## Vascular supply

Blood is supplied to the knee from the genicular arteries and the recurrent branch of the anterior tibial artery (**Figure 9.6**). These vessels are branches of the femoral and popliteal arteries.

## Innervation

The knee is innervated from branches of the femoral, tibial, common peroneal and obturator nerves.

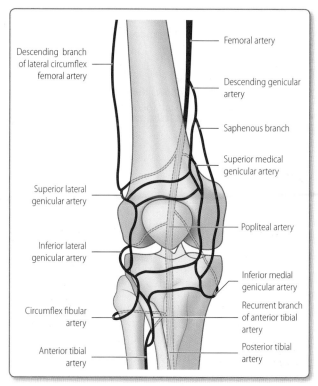

**Figure 9.6** Blood supply to the knee.

## Surface anatomy

The lateral and medial femoral condyles are palpable either side of the patella. When the knee is flexed, the joint line is palpable horizontally between the femoral and tibial condyles. The patella and quadriceps tendon can be palpated in both flexion and extension. The medial and lateral collateral ligaments can be palpated either side of the knee over their bony insertions.

# 9.3 Examination

### Key signs

Key signs to assess for include varus or valgus deformity, swelling/effusion, reduced range of movement and an inability to straight leg raise.

### Examination sequence

Examination of the knee follows the system of 'Look, feel and move' from proximal to distal, followed by tests of function. Neurological signs are then sought, and pulses and capillary refill checked.

### Look

- Look for swelling
- Look for bruising
- Is there any erythema?
- Is there any deformity, either valgus or varus?

### Feel

- Is the knee warm compared with the other knee?
- Palpate for an effusion with a patellar tap (**Figure 9.7**) or sweep test
- Palpate for bony tenderness over the joint line and patella

### Move

- Extend and flex the knee joint; what is the range of movement? (The normal range of movement is 10–140°)
- Can the patient perform a straight leg raise?
- Test collateral ligament stability (**Figure 9.8**)
- Test cruciate ligament stability (**Figure 9.9**)

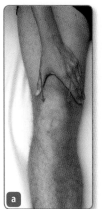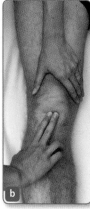

**Figure 9.7** Patellar tap test for knee effusion. (a) Fluid is milked distally from the suprapatellar pouch. Effusion will cause a palpable bulging adjacent to the tendon and (b) a ballotable patella.

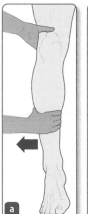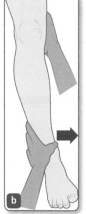

**Figure 9.8** Collateral ligament stability testing: (a) medial stress and (b) lateral stress

## Function

- Test the nerves and feel the dorsalis pedis and posterior tibial pulses
- Can the patient weight-bear?
- Assess gait

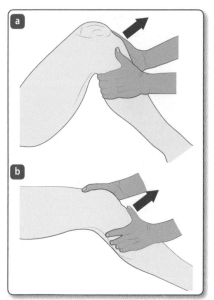

**Figure 9.9** Cruciate ligament testing: (a) anterior draw test and (b) Lachman test.

## 9.4 Patellar fractures

Patella fractures account for approximately 1 in 100 orthopaedic fractures.

### Epidemiology

Patellar fractures are most commonly encountered in men more frequently than women and in the age range 18–50 years.

### Causes

This type of fracture is usually caused by indirect trauma. Sudden contraction of the quadriceps usually leads to a transverse fracture. A similar mechanism of sudden contraction of the quadriceps muscle can cause rupture of either the patellar ligament or quadriceps tendon. Direct trauma, for example from a fall on to the knee, usually produces more complex fracture patterns (**Figure 9.10**).

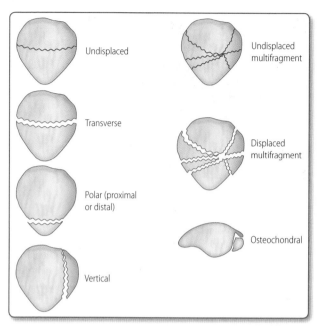

**Figure 9.10** Fracture patterns of the patella.

## Clinical features

Patients with patellar fracture typically present with pain and swelling of the knee and difficulty standing or weight-bearing. Bruising is usually present and they may have evidence of a graze or wound if they have fallen directly onto the knee. Patients are usually unable to perform a straight leg raise. Patellar fractures are normally unilateral.

## Investigations

Anteroposterior and lateral radiographs of the knee are required, and show a fracture and the degree of displacement, and also whether the fracture is simple or complex with comminution (**Figure 9.11**).

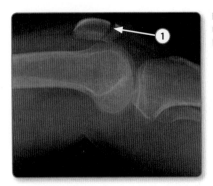

**Figure 9.11** Lateral radiograph showing a patellar fracture ①.

## Management

**Conservative management** For non-displaced fractures with an intact extensor mechanism, a knee splint or cylinder cast is usually applied and the patient allowed to weight-bear as pain allows. As the fracture heals, the splint or cast is replaced with a hinged knee brace. The brace enables them to start actively flexing, extending and strengthening the quadriceps muscles.

**Surgical management** Surgery is indicated in cases of loss of active extension, a displaced fracture, an open fracture or intra-articular displacement. Tension band wires (**Figure 9.13**), cerclage wires or even multiple screws and wires may be used if the fracture is comminuted.

After the operation, the knee is placed in a splint. If the fracture is severely comminuted, the patient may also be immobilised. If not, partial to full weight-bearing is encouraged over the next 6 weeks.

Patellectomy may be indicated in cases of severely comminuted fracture. However, it is associated with very poor long-term outcomes, so is considered only for the worst cases of patellar fracture.

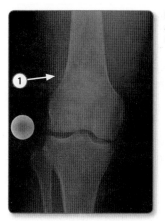

**Figure 9.12** Anteroposterior showing a bipartite patella. ① Secondary unfused ossification centre.

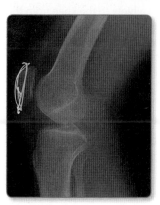

**Figure 9.13** Lateral radiograph showing tension band wiring of a patella.

**Complications** These are:
- failure of fixation
- refracture
- non-union
- patellofemoral osteoarthritis
- reduced knee movement
- extensor lag or loss of extensor strength
- instability

## 9.5 Patellar dislocation

Patella dislocations can be acute and secondary to significant trauma, but more commonly they are due to the patient's anatomical factors. Some patients will have recurrent dislocations and have regular presentations to their GP or emergency department.

### Epidemiology

Patellar dislocations are most often encountered in young adults, particularly women, and patients with hypermobility or connective tissue disorders.

### Causes

Patellar dislocations, like patellar fractures, are caused by either indirect injury, for example sudden muscular contraction, or direct trauma, for example from a blow to the knee from the side. People with hypermobile joints can have frequent dislocations, which occur easily, with very little pressure. Congenital abnormalities of the patella also increase the risk of dislocation.

### Clinical features

The most common clinical features of patellar dislocation are:
- extreme pain
- knee swelling
- deformity
- inability to flex the knee
- inability to stand or weight-bear

### Investigations

Anteroposterior and lateral radiographs of the knee are required. Lateral dislocation is most common; it is associated with osteochondral fracture in up to 5% of cases. The osteochondral fracture is may only be apparent if it is present on a skyline view.

> ## Guiding principle
>
> The Beighton score is used to quantify joint hypermobility and laxity (**Table 9.1**). A score of > 6 out of 9 indicates hypermobility. Patients with hypermobility are at risk of recurrent dislocations.

| Joint | Finding | Score |
|-------|---------|-------|
| Left little finger | Passive dorsiflexion > 90 | 1 |
| Right little finger | Passive dorsiflexion > 90 | 1 |
| Left thumb | Passive palmarflexion to flexor aspect of forearm | 1 |
| Right thumb | Passive palmarflexion to flexor aspect of forearm | 1 |
| Left elbow | Hyperextends beyond 10° | 1 |
| Right elbow | Hyperextends beyond 10° | 1 |
| Left knee | Hyperextends beyond 10° | 1 |
| Right knee | Hyperextends beyond 10° | 1 |
| Spine | On forward flexion, palms and hands can rest on floor | 1 |

Table 9.1 The Beighton score for joint hypermobility.

## Management

Reduction is attempted in the emergency department, and with adequate analgesia is normally successful. If reduction fails, manipulation under anaesthesia in the operating theatre is required. Firm lateral pressure is needed with the knee in extension. A radiograph is obtained to confirm reduction. A skyline view is helpful to detect any osteochondral fracture.

Immobilisation in a cylinder cast or cricket pad splint keeps the knee in extension for a minimum of 2 weeks; it is then reviewed in the fracture clinic. At this point, a referral to physiotherapy is normally made for exercises to slowly improve flexion and to strengthen the quadriceps. Surgery is normally considered only for recurrent dislocations, and is carried out by a soft tissue knee surgeon.

## 9.6 Tibial plateau fractures

The tibial plateau is one of the main load-bearing areas of the body, so it is important that fractures of the tibial plateau are not missed. Because the articular surface of the knee joint is involved in these injuries, patients need to be aware that they will have an increased chance of developing arthritic changes in the knee at an earlier than normal stage in their lives.

## Epidemiology

Tibial plateau fractures are more common in elderly patients. In younger patients, they are usually not isolated injuries but part of polytrauma or open injuries. Associated injury to the soft tissues is present in up to 90% of cases of tibial plateau fractures.

## Causes

This type of fracture occurs because of varus or valgus stress combined with axial loading. Various mechanisms of injury lead to different fracture patterns.

- In older patients, poor bone quality means that much less force is required to produce a tibial plateau fracture; it can be caused by an accidental fall
- In younger patients, increased force is required to produce this fracture; it is often the result of a road traffic accident or other high energy mechanism

## Clinical features

Tibial plateau fractures present with:

- knee swelling
- pain
- inability to weight-bear, or difficulty weight-bearing
- ligamentous injuries of the knee or other associated soft tissue injuries, so it is important to assess the stability of the knee

A full trauma survey is required if the fracture is a result of high-energy trauma. Neurovascular examination is also needed, taking particular note of distal pulses and the common peroneal nerve, which can be stretched, resulting in neuropraxia. In addition, the risk of compartment syndrome must be considered in high-energy injuries.

## Investigations

Anteroposterior and lateral radiographs of the knee are required initially, but it may also be possible to obtain specific lateral and medial plateau views. CT is the preferred investigation for further assessment of a tibial plateau fracture; it is used to gauge the degree of depression and thereby help determine whether conservative or surgical management is required. Meniscal injuries are associated with tibial plateau fracture, so MRI scans are needed to evaluate this.

## Management

The Schatzker classification is the best-known system for categorising tibial plateau fractures (**Table 9.2**). Classification helps guide management. Type II fractures are the most common (**Figure 9.14**). Types IV–VI are normally associated with high-energy trauma.

**Conservative management**  This approach is used for patients with non-displaced or minimally displaced (usually < 2–10 mm) fractures, and for the very elderly, bedbound or unwell with multiple medical co-morbidities. A cylinder cast or hinged knee brace is applied. Only partial weight bearing is allowed for the first 6–8 weeks, before progressing to full weight-bearing. Patients will undergo physiotherapy, particularly exercises to strengthen the quadriceps and thereby increase the active range of movement.

**Surgical management**  Surgery is required for displaced fractures, open fractures and fractures associated with vascular injury. The aims are to reconstruct the articular surface and realign the tibia. Various methods are used, depending on the state of the soft tissue.

- If there is significant soft tissue injury, spanning external fixation is used
- If there is no soft tissue damage, Kirschner wires, tension band wires, screws or plates are used, depending on the fracture configuration and surgical preference

Bone graft may be used if there is a significant depression injury. Because of the high incidence of meniscal injuries in cases of tibial plateau fracture, arthroscopy is occasionally also used intraoperatively to assess the articular surface, menisci and cruciate ligaments. A splint is used postoperatively. Postop-

| Type | Description of fracture pattern | |
|------|-------------------------------|---|
| I | Lateral split | |
| II | Lateral split with depression | |
| III | Lateral depression | |
| IV | Medial fracture | |
| V | Bicondylar fracture | |
| VI | Fracture with metaphyseal–diaphyseal separation | |

**Table 9.2** Schatzker classification of tibial plateau fractures.

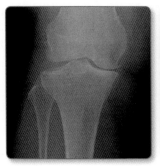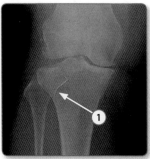

**Figure 9.14** Anteroposterior radiograph of the right knee, showing a Schatzker type II tibial plateau fracture. On the second image, the fracture line has been demarcated.

erative weight bearing status can vary depending on fracture pattern and surgical fixation. **Figure 9.15** shows plate fixation of a Schatzker type II fracture.

**Complications** Potential complications of tibial plateau fracture are:
- deep vein thrombosis or pulmonary embolism
- infection
- compartment syndrome
- arthrofibrosis
- osteoarthritis
- peroneal nerve injury
- popliteal artery injury
- malunion and non-union
- loose bodies in the knee joint

## 9.7 Tibial shaft fractures

Tibial shaft fractures occur in the diaphysis of the tibia. They occur at any point in the tibial diaphysis and can extend into the knee, or more commonly, the ankle joint.

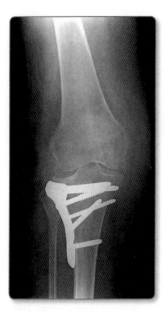

**Figure 9.15** Anteroposterior radiograph of the right knee, showing plate fixation of a Schatzker type II fracture.

## Epidemiology

Tibial shaft fractures are the most common long bone fracture and account for up to 4% of all fractures.

## Causes

The two main mechanisms of injury are low energy, torsional injuries that lead to a spiral fracture configuration, and high energy fractures that more commonly lead to a transverse fracture pattern. These high energy fractures can also be associated with fibula fractures and soft tissue or open injuries.

## Clinical features

Patients present with pain and inability to weight bear. On examination they may have a deformity, soft tissue injury, open wounds or evidence of compartment syndrome, making careful neurovascular examination crucial.

### Investigations
Anteroposterior and lateral radiographs are required and CT can be organised to assess the fracture pattern in more detail. CT can also help with surgical planning and clarify any concerns about intra-articular extension.

### Management
Tibial shaft fractures are treated both conservatively and surgically.

### Conservative management
Closed lower energy injuries with minimal displacement can be treated with a plaster cast and immobilisation. Less than 5° of varus–valgus angulation, <10° of sagittal plane angulation, <1 cm shortening or <10° of rotational malalignment are all acceptable measures for conservative treatment. The patient will be non-weight bearing in a plaster cast for a minimum of 6 weeks and will require regular fracture clinic review to check there is no further displacement or loss of position.

### Surgical management
The majority of tibial shaft fractures are treated surgically as patients can potentially weight bear immediately. The surgical options are external fixation (for open injuries or fractures with significant associated soft tissue injuries); intramedullary nail and open reduction; and internal fixation with a combination of plates or screws.

## 9.8 Distal femoral fractures
Distal femoral fractures are classed as fractures within the distal third of the femur. They can involve the articular surface.

### Epidemiology
The incidence of femoral fractures has a bimodal distribution, peaking at about 24 and 65 years of age.

### Causes
In the young, these injuries tend to be associated with high-speed blunt trauma, such as that from a fall from height or a

road traffic accident. In the elderly, distal femoral fractures are associated with low-energy trauma and poor bone quality.

## Clinical features

Patients with distal femoral fracture present with:
- pain
- inability to weight-bear
- swelling and bruising
- deformity

The possibility of compartment syndrome must be considered.

## Investigations

Anteroposterior and lateral radiographs are obtained. If the fracture involves the knee joint, CT is also indicated to aid in preoperative planning. **Figure 9.16** shows a high-energy transverse distal femoral fracture.

## Management

Management of this type of fracture depends on whether the injury is open or closed, the degree of displacement, and the

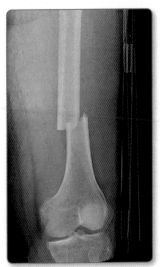

**Figure 9.16** Anteroposterior radiograph of the distal femur showing a transverse fracture of the distal third of the femur.

status of the patient before the injury, in terms of mobility and comorbidities.

**Conservative management** This consists of use of a hinged brace for 6 weeks, with no weight-bearing. This is suitable for patients with a non-displaced fracture and who have limited mobility, significant comorbidities, or both.

**Surgical management** Surgery is considered for patients with displaced or intra-articular fracture. Open reduction and internal fixation, using an intramedullary nail or plates and screws, is indicated.

**Complications** The complications of distal femoral fracture are:
- non-union or malunion
- vascular injury (because of the proximity of the popliteal artery)
- irritation from metalwork
- knee stiffness
- gait disturbance

# 9.9 Quadriceps and patellar tendon injuries

Tendon injuries are most commonly secondary to eccentric loading of the knee extensor mechanism. Quadriceps tendon injuries are more common than injuries to the patella tendon, and can be partial or complete.

## Epidemiology
Ruptures of the extensor mechanism are more common in men aged > 40 years. Poor vasculature is a risk factor for extensor tendon rupture, so it is associated with diabetes, renal failure, use of cortisone injections and rheumatoid arthritis. There are similar risk factors for patella tendon rupture but patients are usually < 40 years.

## Causes
Quadriceps and patellar tendon injuries usually occur as a consequence of a fall with the knee in extension, or blunt trauma.

### Clinical features

Patients with these injuries present with:

- pain
- haemarthrosis and associated joint swelling
- inability to perform a straight leg raise (in cases of complete rupture)
- inability to weight-bear or walk
- mobile patella or a palpable defect above the patella

### Investigations

Anteroposterior and lateral radiographs of the knee are obtained. A radiograph of the contralateral side is also usually obtained for comparison. If there is any doubt, ultrasound, MRI (**Figure 9.17**) or both are useful for confirmation; they can also help to determine whether the tear is full or partial.

### Management

Management can vary depending on whether the rupture or tear is partial or complete.

**Conservative management** This approach is indicated for patients with an incomplete tear and a preserved extensor mechanism, and for those who are not well enough for surgery. It consists of holding the leg in extension in a brace for 6 weeks.

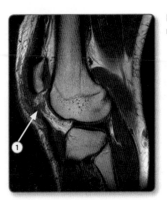

**Figure 9.17** Sagittal MRI scan showing rupture of the patellar tendon ①.

**Surgical management**  Surgical reattachment of the tendon is indicated for complete ruptures. The leg also has to be held in extension in a brace for about 6 weeks. The patient can weight-bear providing the leg is in extension.

**Complications**  Potential complications are a reduced range of movement, weakness and knee stiffness. Rerupture can also occur.

## 9.10 Soft tissue injuries

Soft tissue injuries of the knee are a common presentation to the emergency department and vary in type and severity.

The most commonly injured ligament is the anterior cruciate ligament.

The medial meniscus is injured more frequently than the lateral meniscus.

### Causes

Twisting injuries damage the ligaments, the menisci or both. Blunt trauma can result in multiple areas of soft tissue injury, especially when associated with dislocation of the knee.

### Clinical features

Patients with soft tissue injuries of the knee present with:
- pain
- swelling
- haemarthrosis
- reduced range of movement
- inability to weight-bear

Meniscal tears occasionally cause locking or clicking of the knee joint. The joint swelling associated with meniscal tears is commonly intermittent. The integrity of the ligaments is tested by stressing the joint during examination. A history of a 'pop' or 'click' followed by massive, tense, painful haemarthrosis strongly suggests rupture of the anterior cruciate ligament.

In any ligament injury, the knee may be too swollen initially for examination to yield any useful information. If this is the case, it is prudent to splint the knee and ask the patient to return in 2 weeks for examination.

### Investigations

Anteroposterior and lateral radiographs are required. MRI is carried out if there is any doubt about the nature of the injury. **Figure 9.18** shows an injury to the anterior cruciate ligament.

### Management

> ### Clinical insight
>
> A Segond fracture, an avulsion fracture of the lateral tibial plateau, is pathognomonic for rupture of an anterior cruciate ligament (see **Figure 9.19**).

**Conservative management** This consists of rest, the application of ice, elevation, use of non-steroidal anti-inflammatory drugs and physiotherapy. Ligamentous injuries can be treated non-operatively, or reviewed at a later date if the patient has ongoing symptoms.

**Surgical management** Operative management for meniscal injuries includes partial meniscectomy or repair.

The anterior cruciate ligament is more commonly reconstructed if the patient is young or an active older individual. The patient's functional level helps determine the appropriate management option. All surgery for soft tissue injuries of the knee (apart from multi-ligament injuries with associated

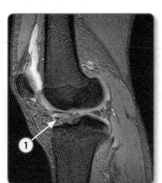

**Figure 9.18** Sagittal MRI showing a tear through the anterior cruciate ligament ①, which has been avulsed from its origin at the anterior medial tibia, with loss of the normal 'bundle' morphology.

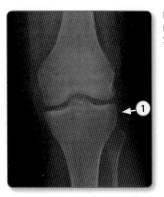

**Figure 9.19** Anteroposterior radiograph of the knee, showing a Segond fracture ①.

fractures, dislocations or acutely locked knees) is often performed as elective surgery after a period of rehabilitation.

## 9.11 Osteoarthritis

Osteoarthritis is a chronic, progressive, degenerative condition that affects synovial joints. It results in loss of articular cartilage and hypertrophic bone changes.

### Epidemiology

Osteoarthritis is more common in women than men, and its prevalence increases with age. The hips, knees and hands are the most common sites for osteoarthritis.

> **Clinical insight**
>
> A Pellegrini–Stieda lesion is ossification of the medial collateral ligament. It indicates a possible associated injury to the medial collateral ligament (**Figure 9.20**).

### Causes

The cause is unknown. However, risk factors include obesity, trauma and muscle weakness.

### Clinical features

Joints are painful, swollen and stiff, especially early in the morning. These symptoms ease as the day progresses. On examination, there is usually reduced range of motion, joint effusions and joint malalignment.

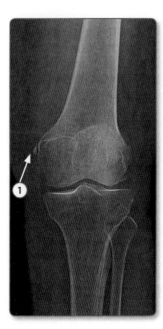

**Figure 9.20** Anteroposterior radiograph of the knee, showing Pellegrini–Stieda lesion ①.

## Guiding principles

The four key radiological findings of osteoarthritis are:

- joint space narrowing
- subchondral sclerosis
- subchondral cysts
- osteophytes

### Investigations

Anteroposterior and lateral radiographs of the affected joint are required. **Figure 9.21** shows osteoarthritis of the knee.

### Management

**Conservative management** This is always tried in cases of osteoarthritis. Options include walking aids, anti-inflammatory medications, analgesia, weight loss and joint injections. Outcomes are measured in terms of function and pain.

**Surgical management** Surgery is reserved for when pain, reduced function or both are significantly reducing a patient's

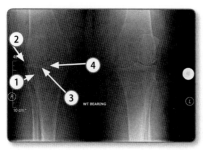

**Figure 9.21**
Anteroposterior radiograph radiograph showing osteoarthritis of the right knee, with loss of joint space ①, subchondral sclerosis ②, osteophytes ③ and cysts ④.

quality of life. It includes joint replacement and in most cases has a very good outcome. After hip or knee replacement, the outcome is good or excellent in 95% of patients.

# 9.12 Knee dislocation

Dislocation of the knee is rare. However, it is a highly serious orthopaedic emergency and should not be trivialised. This injury should be urgently referred to the senior registrar on call. Knee dislocations are associated with vascular injuries and multi-ligament injuries of the knee.

## Epidemiology

Due to the high energy nature of this injury it is more common in patients <50 years, and also in patients with increased body mass index following a fall.

## Causes

Knee dislocations are most likely to result from high-energy road traffic accidents, for example when a knee hits the dashboard, because significant soft tissue injury or disruption of all the ligaments is usually required for the knee to dislocate. The injuries occasionally happen during sport. Knee dislocation is not a benign injury.

## Clinical features

Patients present with:
- deformity of the knee, if it does not reduce spontaneously

- pain
- effusion and swelling
- instability
- ligamentous laxity injuries of the knee

The popliteal vessels are extremely vulnerable to injury during dislocation. Therefore it is crucial to check and document the distal pulses, i.e. the dorsalis pedis and posterior tibial. Significant vascular injury is present in up to 15% of knee dislocations.

A thorough distal neurological examination is also required. The common peroneal nerve is the nerve most likely to be injured in knee dislocations.

## Investigations

After reduction, anterior and lateral radiographs of the knee are obtained to confirm reduction and to ensure that no other fractures are present. This is necessary because dislocations can have associated fractures of the tibia or fibula.

> ### Clinical insight
>
> If the knee has not reduced spontaneously, immediate reduction is carried out before investigations are arranged. Vascular status before and after reduction must be documented.

Up to 50% of knee dislocations have associated injury to the popliteal artery. If the distal pulse is absent or diminished, or if the ankle–brachial pressure index is < 0.9, urgent CT angiogram or in theatre angiography is requested and vascular surgeons are notified. In cases of injury to the popliteal artery, immediate surgical exploration is indicated and revascularisation should be carried out within 8 h. A popliteal injury is suspected in all knee dislocations, because it is limb-threatening.

## Management

Immediate reduction is required if the knee has not already reduced spontaneously.

**Conservative management** This consists of immobilisation of the knee in a splint or plaster to hold the knee in extension for ≥ 6 weeks.

**Surgical management**  Surgery is required if the knee is unstable and in cases of open wounds or vascular injury. Depending on the condition of the soft tissues, either external fixators or open reduction and internal fixation is used. If vascular injury is present, the vascular team should be involved as soon as possible, because any delay can reduce the likelihood of survival of the limb.

Delayed ligamentous reconstruction may be required to formally stabilise the knee at a later date, usually once the swelling has reduced. This may be done as a staged procedure.

**Complications**  Possible complications of knee dislocation are:
- popliteal artery injury
- peroneal nerve injury or neuropraxia
- reduced range of motion and knee stiffness
- ligamentous injury

# Foot and ankle

The foot and ankle are a complex series of joints and levers funtioning as a unit and adapting to changing terrain, enabling us to walk in different environments.

The gait cycle begins when one foot contacts the ground at the heel. The portion of the foot in contact with the ground progresses forwards until toe-off, when the toe rises from the ground. The foot then swings forwards before hitting the ground again, marking the start of the next cycle.

The complexity of movement achievable by the foot and ankle allows humans to carry out diverse activities, such as ballet and football. However, these movements place demands on the foot and ankle that can cause trivial or serious injuries.

## 10.1 Clinical scenario

### Acute calf pain

#### Background

A 41-year-old man, while playing squash after work, experienced severe pain at the back of his calf when he pushed off rapidly with his left foot to get into position. It felt as if he had been hit in the back of the leg with a racquet. He was able to walk uncomfortably but was unable to continue playing. Therefore he went to the nearest emergency department.

#### History

The patient has no significant medical history.

#### Examination

Inspection finds swelling of the left ankle posteriorly.

> **Clinical insight**
>
> The calf squeeze test, also known as Simmonds' or Thompson's test, must be carried out when an Achilles tendon is suspected. Record whether the ankle did or did not plantar flex on squeezing the calf. Absence of plantar flexion implies that the Achilles tendon has been ruptured. After 2 weeks, the test becomes far less reliable; by this time, scar tissue has reduced the gap in the ruptured tendon, so movement may be elicited by squeezing.

There is no bony tenderness, but the patient has tenderness within the Achilles tendon, with a palpable gap. The calf squeeze test finds an absence of plantar flexion of the ankle on the affected side.

### Differential diagnosis
Possible causes of the patient's symptoms are:
- Achilles tendon rupture
- gastrocnemius or soleus tear
- ankle fracture
- Achilles tendinopathy

An acute Achilles tendon rupture is diagnosed. The diagnosis is largely clinical; rupture must be considered in anyone presenting with sudden and severe pain to the Achilles, especially after high exertion. The patient is admitted for repair.

### Investigations
Ultrasound is a quick and reliable investigation to confirm the diagnosis of acute rupture.

## 10.2 Anatomy
The foot comprises 26 bones and is divided into the forefoot, mid-foot and hindfoot (**Figure 10.1, 10.2** and **10.3**). The ankle consists of three bones: the distal aspect of the tibia and fibula, the bony protuberances of which form the medial and lateral malleoli, respectively and the talus, which sits within this mortise.

### Ligaments
The talus is connected to the tibia and fibula by ligaments (**Figures 10.1** and **10.2**). The main ligament on the medial side of the ankle (**Figure 10.2**) is the deltoid ligament which has multiple parts and is split into superficial and deep. The ligaments on the lateral side (**Figure 10.1**) are made up of three separate parts: the anterior talofibular ligament, the calcaneofibular ligament and the posterior talofibular ligament.

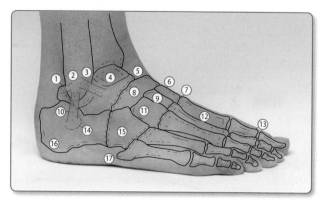

**Figure 10.1** Lateral view of bones and ligaments of the foot. ① Posterior talofibular ligament, ② lateral malleolus, ③ anterior talofibular ligament, ④ body of talus, ⑤ head of talus and transverse tarsal joint line (Chopart's joint) (orange), ⑥ medial cuneiform, ⑦ tarsometatarsal joint line (orange), ⑧ navicular, ⑨ intermediate cuneiform, ⑩ calcaneofibular ligament, ⑪ lateral cuneiform, ⑫ 1st metatarsal, ⑬ phalanges of digit 1 (proximal and distal), ⑭ fibular trochlea, ⑮ cuboid, ⑯ calcaneal tuberosity, ⑰ tuberosity of 5th metatarsal.

**Note:** ligaments 1, 3 and 10 collectively form the lateral collateral ligament.

## Vascular supply

The blood supply of the foot (**Figures 10.4** and **10.5**) comes from three main arteries: the peroneal, posterior tibial and anterior tibial arteries. It is a branch of the anterior tibial artery which can be palpated over the dorsum of the foot just lateral to the extensor hallucis longus tendon and the dorsalis pedis pulse.

## Innervation

The main nerves to the foot are the tibial nerve (dividing into the medial and lateral plantar nerves), sural nerve, deep peroneal nerve, superficial peroneal nerve and saphenous nerve (see **Figures 10.4** and **10.5**). Knowledge of these nerves is essential when assessing for neurological deficit (**Table 10.1**).

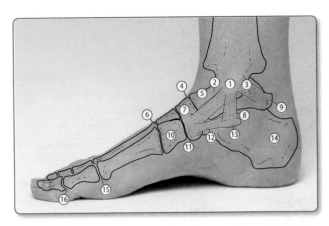

**Figure 10.2** Bones and ligaments of the medial right foot. ① Medial malleolus, ② anterior tibiotalar ligament, ③ posterior tibiotalar ligament, ④ transverse tarsal joint line (Chopart's Joint) (orange), ⑤ head of talus, ⑥ tarsometatarsal joint line (orange), ⑦ tibionavicular ligament, ⑧ tibiocalcaneal ligament, ⑨ posterior process of talus, ⑩ medial cuneiform, ⑪ navicular tuberosity, ⑫ calcaneonavicular/spring ligament, ⑬ sustentaculum tali, ⑭ calcaneus, ⑮ first metatarsophalangeal joint, ⑯ interphalangeal joint of digit 1.
**Note:** ligaments 2, 3, 7 and 8 collectively form the medial collateral (deltoid) ligament.

### Surface anatomy
Many features of the bones and joints of the foot can be identified on the dorsum or sides of the foot by palpation during examination (**Figures 10.1, 10.2** and **10.3**).

## 10.3 Examination

### Key signs
Key signs to assess for include swelling, bruising, deformity, tenderness and instability.

### Examination sequence
Examination follows a system of 'Look, feel and move', starting proximally and moving distally, followed by tests of function.

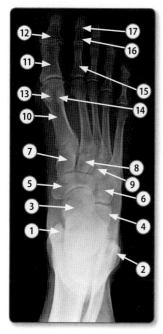

**Figure 10.3** (1) Medial malleolus (tibia), (2) lateral malleolus (fibula), (3) talus, (4) calcaneus, (5) navicular, (6) cuboid, (7) medial cuneiform, (8) middle (intermediate) cuneiform, (9) lateral cuneiform, (10) 1st metatarsal, (11) proximal phalanx of hallux, (12) distal phalanx of hallux, (13) tibial (medial) sesamoid, (14) fibula (lateral) sesamoid, (15) proximal phalanx of 2nd toe, (16) middle phalanx of 2nd toe, (17) distal phalanx of 2nd toe.

### Look

- Observe for swelling and bruising – where is it located?
- Is the foot pointing in the same direction as the knee on the same side?
- Is there any deformity?
- Are the toes aligned?
- Note the skin colour and any breaks in the skin

### Feel

- Palpate for bony tenderness at the malleoli
- Palpate the anterior joint line of the ankle
- Palpate the bones of the foot
- Palpate the Achilles tendon for tenderness and discontinuity
- Palpate the lateral ankle ligaments and deltoid ligament

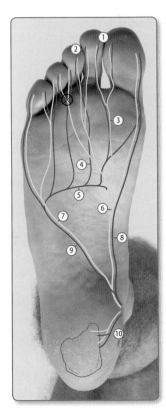

**Figure 10.4** Neurovasculature of the plantar foot. ① Plantar digital nerves, ② plantar digital arteries, ③ common plantar nerve, ④ common plantar artery, ⑤ deep plantar arterial arch, ⑥ medial plantar nerve, ⑦ lateral plantar nerve, ⑧ medial plantar artery, ⑨ lateral plantar artery, ⑩ medial calcaneal artery and nerve, ⊗ site of painful Morton's neuroma (perineural fibrosis).

### Move

- Assess ankle joint movement (**Figure 10.6**)
- Assess subtalar joint movement
- Assess midtarsal joint movement
- Assess foot and toes movement (**Figure 10.7**)

### Function

- Test the nerves (see Innervation section above) and feel the dorsalis pedis and posterior tibial pulses (**Table 10.1**)
- Can the patient weight-bear?

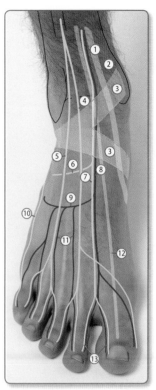

**Figure 10.5** Neurovasculature of the dorsal foot. ① Anterior tibial artery, ② tibialis anterior tendon, ③ inferior extensor retinaculum, ④ medial dorsal cutaneous nerve, ⑤ intermediate dorsal cutaneous nerve, ⑥ lateral branch of deep peroneal nerve, ⑦ medial branch of deep peroneal nerve, ⑧ dorsalis pedis artery, ⑨ arcuate artery, ⑩ lateral dorsal cutaneous nerve, ⑪ dorsal metatarsal arteries, ⑫ extensor hallucis longus tendon, ⑬ dorsal digital arteries and nerves.

| Nerve | Nerve roots | Sensation innervation | Motor test |
|---|---|---|---|
| Saphenous | L3 and L4 | Medial malleolus | Sensory only |
| Deep peroneal | L4 and L5 | 1st web space | Toe and foot dorsiflexion |
| Superficial peroneal | L5 and S1 | Dorsum of foot | Foot eversion |
| Tibial (medial, lateral plantar and calcaneal branches) | S1 and S2 | Plantar surface of foot | Foot inversion and foot plantar flexion |
| Sural | S1 and S2 | Lateral border of foot | Sensory only |

**Table 10.1** Nerves of the foot and ankle.

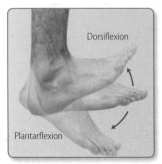

**Figure 10.6** Ankle plantarflexion (45–55°) and dorsiflexion (15–20°).

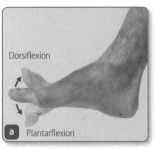

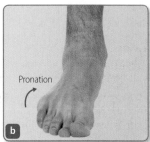

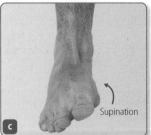

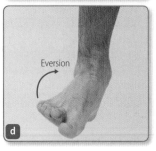

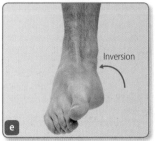

**Figure 10.7** Foot and toe movements. (a) Dorsiflexion/plantarflexion, (b) pronation, (c) supination, (d) eversion, (15-20º), (e) inversion (35º).

## 10.4 Ankle fractures

An ankle fracture can involve the:
- lateral malleolus (distal fibula)
- medial malleolus (medial tibia)
- posterior part (posterior malleolus) of the distal tibia

Presenting symptoms are similar to those of ankle ligamentous injuries but are usually more severe. Ankle fractures occasionally present late; if patients can weight-bear, they may not realise the ankle is broken. They are frequently associated with dislocations.

> ### Clinical insight
>
> Ankle fractures can occur in the absence of significant trauma, especially in older patients with osteoporosis. To avoid missed diagnoses, radiographs are obtained in cases of doubt.

### Epidemiology

Ankle fractures are common, with an incidence of up to 200 fractures per 100,000 people each year. The incidence is increasing in the western world because of greater participation in sport, the growing elderly population and the rise in obesity.

### Causes

The mechanism of injury is commonly a fall or twisting injury. Other causes include direct trauma and repetitive loading, which can occur when a person suddenly takes up running, for example.

### Clinical features

The ankle is likely to be swollen. Bony tenderness is present on the lateral or medial malleolus, or both. There is occasionally a deformity, commonly the foot facing sideways (laterally) as a result of associated dislocation.

> ### Clinical insight
>
> A Maisonneuve fracture is a spiral fracture of the proximal fibula caused by external rotation injury and associated with rupture of the syndesmosis, deltoid ligament and interosseous membrane. It is easily missed, very unstable and must be treated promptly and appropriately to avoid mismanagement and associated complications.
>
> Look out for a Maisonneuve fracture in patients with a high fibular fracture, increased medial space or widening of the syndesmosis without an obvious ankle fracture on radiography. Clinically there willl be tenderness around the knee at the proximal fibula.

*Lateral aspect of the knee (fibula head)*

## Clinical insight

If an ankle is found to be obviously dislocated on initial assessment, reduction must be carried out as soon as possible – do not wait for a radiograph.

## Clinical insight

The Ottawa ankle rules (**Figure 10.8**) are used to decide whether a radiograph of the ankle is necessary after an ankle injury. A radiograph is required if there is:

- pain in the malleolar region and bony tenderness along the distal posterior edge of the tibia or tip of the medial malleolus;
- bony tenderness along the distal posterior edge of the fibula or tip of the lateral malleolus; or
- an inability to weight-bear

If there is no bony tenderness in the areas described, a fracture is very unlikely.

The knee and whole length of the fibula must be assessed for tenderness. With some ankle fracture patterns, for example the Maisonneuve fracture, the fibular fracture is closer to the knee. Neurovascular compromise is occasionally present.

If the fracture is open, the site and size of the wound are assessed and the wound checked for contamination. The choice of management of even benign open fractures can depend on the nature of the wound.

### Investigations

Anteroposterior and lateral radiographs of the ankle are required as a minimum. If further information is needed

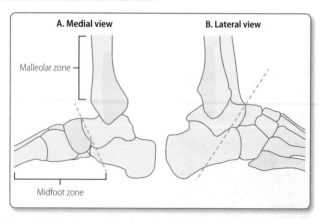

**A. Medial view**

**B. Lateral view**

Malleolar zone

Midfoot zone

**Figure 10.8** The Ottowa ankle rules. Radiographs are required if there is bony tenderness in the blue-shaded areas (see box).

about the ankle mortise, a mortise view is obtained (**Figure 10.9**). This is a view of the ankle with the leg internally rotated by 15°. If there is no fibular fracture at the ankle but bony tenderness around the knee, an anteroposterior view of the knee is required.

Examination of the radiograph includes:

- inspection for fractures of the lateral, medial and posterior malleolus
- assessment of the degree of displacement
- determination of the level of the fracture line

The relation between the talus and the medial and lateral malleoli is assessed on the anteroposterior view. The joint line often referred to as the mortise should be equal at all levels and is generally a space of 2–4 mm. Disruption of the mortise usually indicates displacement of the fracture with instability.

Fractures of both the lateral malleolus and the medial malleolus are known as bimalleolar fractures. Fractures of the lateral, medial and posterior malleoli are known as trimalleolar fractures. As a general rule, the more bones broken in the ankle, the more displaced and unstable the fracture.

**Classification** Systems commonly used to categorise ankle fractures include the Danis–Weber classification (often known as the Weber classification), which is based on the level of fracture at the distal fibula (**Table 10.2** and **Figures 10.10** and **10.11**), and the Lauge–Hansen classification, based on the

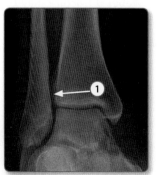

Figure 10.9 'Mortise' view radiograph of ankle ① the normal tibiofibular overlap is >1mm on the mortise view.

mechanism of injury. The Lauge–Hansen classification gives first the position of the foot at the time of injury and then the force applied to the ankle, for example supination–external rotation. A small proportion of ankle fractures are unclassifiable.

## Management

The aim of ankle fracture treatment is restoration of articular anatomy and fibular rotation and length. Preservation of the articular surfaces prevents future complications such as post-traumatic arthritis.

**Emergency management**  Fracture dislocations (**Figure 10.11**) are an emergency situation. The diagnosis is clinical, and obtaining radiographs should not delay reduction. A dislocation can compromise blood supply to the foot and skin. Prompt reduction of the articular surfaces and splintage mitigate complications, including post-traumatic arthritis.

**Conservative management**  Isolated non-displaced medial malleolar fractures, Weber A fractures and non-displaced Weber B fractures are likely to be stable. There is a chance that an undisplaced Weber B fracture may be

> ## Guiding principle
>
> A stable fracture is one that will not displace under physiological load, i.e. the load imposed when standing or walking. An obviously displaced fracture is likely to be unstable. Less displaced fractures are more difficult to assess.
>
> The key to stability is the integrity of the medial structures. A fracture of the lateral malleolus with bruising and swelling, along with tenderness to palpation at the medial side, may indicate a medial (deltoid) ligament injury, which can predict an unstable injury.

| Type | Level of fracture |
|------|-------------------|
| A | Below the syndesmosis |
| B | Through the syndesmosis |
| C | Above the syndesmosis |

**Table 10.2** Danis–Weber classification of ankle fractures.

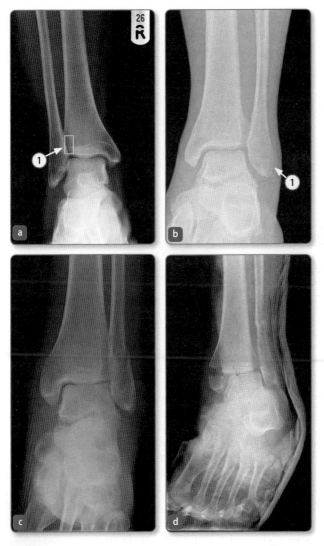

**Figure 10.10** Four different anteroposterior radiographs of ankles (a) ①
indicates the level of the syndesmosis. (b) Weber A fracture. ① Fracture line
indicated below the level of the syndesmosis. (c) A Weber B ankle fracture. (d) A
Weber C ankle fracture with medial malleolus fracture.

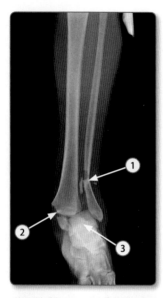

**Figure 10.11** Anteroposterior radiograph of ankle showing a Weber C fracture dislocation of the ankle. There is a fibular fracture ① above the level of the syndesmosis. A medial malleolar fracture ② is also present. The mortise is completely disrupted, with dislocation of the talus ③.

unstable; this may be missed if repeat radiographs of the ankle are not obtained at an early stage, ideally at 1 and 2 weeks. Non-operative treatment is considered for patients who cannot walk or who have more pressing medical problems, for example significant cardiovascular disease.

A below-knee back slab is applied, and a repeat radiograph is done before discharge to check the position of the ankle within the cast. Stable fractures are treated with splinting for the management of pain symptoms. In some patients this may be a walking plaster of Paris cast for 4–6 weeks. After 1 week, radiography is repeated Occasionally reduction is lost and surgical management is required.

**Surgical management** Displacement, talar shift (disruption of the mortise) and dislocation are all indications for surgery. Most ankle fractures are operated on within 24–48 h after injury. Open reduction and internal fixation principally involves applying a plate to the fibula and fixation of the medial malleolus (if necessary), usually with screws (**Figure 10.12**).

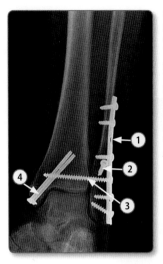

**Figure 10.12** Mortise view of ankle showing an ankle fracture after open reduction and internal fixation. The fibula has been fixed with a plate ① and screws. There is an interfragmentary compression screw ② across the fibular fracture. The syndesmosis has been held with a syndesmosis screw ③. The medial malleolus has been fixed with two compression screws ④.

Patients may be usually discharged with the advice to rest and elevate the leg, then readmitted for planned surgery at a later date. Some patients undergo planned surgery at a later date.

**Complications** The risk of complications increases with increasing levels of fracture complexity. There is a risk of post-traumatic arthritis, even if the articular surface of the ankle appears undisrupted or has been surgically restored.

Common complications include:
- pain or stiffness
- aching in cold weather
- complex regional pain syndrome type 1
- necessity for removal of metalwork at a later date

## 10.5 Pilon fractures

Pilon fractures occur in the distal tibia, within 5 cm of the ankle, and involve the articular surface of the ankle joint. They account for < 10% of all tibial fractures, and 75% of cases have associated fibular fractures.

A pilon fracture implies that a high level of trauma has been sustained by the distal tibia. The joint surface of the tibia at the ankle (plafond) is severely disrupted (**Figure 10.13** and **Figure 10.14**). This type of fracture represents a high-energy injury in

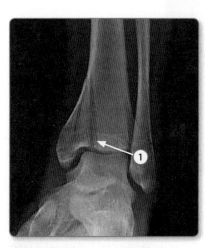

**Figure 10.13**
Anteroposterior radiograph of the ankle, showing a comminuted pilon fracture of the distal tibia ①.

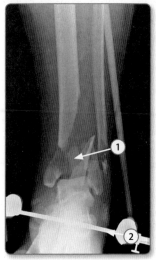

**Figure 10.14** Anteroposterior radiograph of the ankle, showing a high-energy pilon fracture ① with a stabilising cross-ankle external fixator ② applied.

younger patients. There is always significant soft tissue injury, and associated complications are serious.

## Epidemiology

This type of fracture is most common in men aged 25–40 years.

## Causes

The mechanism of injury is high-energy vertical loading that drives the talus into the distal tibia. Pilon fractures are commonly a consequence of motor vehicle accidents or falls from a height. Up to a quarter of these injuries are open fractures (see page 346).

## Clinical features

Clinical features include:

- swelling
- tenderness
- bruising and blistering
- open wounds and soft tissue damage
- vascular injury
- nerve Injury

The patient is assessed for evidence of neurological or vascular injury. Because of the high-energy mechanism of injury of pilon fractures, the spine, hips, knees, feet and contralateral ankle are assessed to exclude concomitant injury. Compartment syndrome should be ruled out (see page 349).

## Investigations

Full-length radiographs of the tibia and fibula, and anteroposterior, lateral and mortise views of the ankle are obtained. A CT scan of the ankle and distal tibia is mandatory to assess the extent of articular involvement and the fracture pattern, and to assist with surgical planning.

## Management

Initial management is first aid: patients are admitted with a below-knee back slab applied and kept non–weight-bearing with the leg elevated. With the back slab in place, the neurovascular status of the limb should be reassessed and documented.

**Conservative management** This is used for stable fractures in patients who:

- are critically ill
- have severe comorbidities
- were unable to walk before the injury
- have no evidence of intra-articular displacement

Conservative management consists of use of a below-knee back slab and remaining non–weight-bearing for 6–8 weeks. Patients are seen within 1 week for review, application of a full plaster of Paris cast and repeat radiography. They are then followed-up weekly for 3–4 weeks.

## Surgical management

Most patients with pilon fractures require surgical management. An external fixator is applied initially to allow the soft tissues to resuscitate, and the swelling to reduce. (**Figure 10.14**). Open reduction and internal fixation is then carried out to restore normal anatomy. Surgery is usually carried out about 2 weeks after the injury.

**Complications** Complications of pilon fractures are usually serious and include:

- chronic ankle pain
- difficulty weight-bearing
- arthritis and/or stiffness from injury to the articular surface

Pilon fractures treated surgically are associated with high levels of complication, reflecting the nature of the injury and the soft tissue insult. The biggest risks are:

- wound breakdown
- infection
- non-union and post-traumatic arthritis

The risks of these complications are much higher in smokers. The risk of non-union is higher if there is significant disruption between the metaphysis and the diaphysis. Often, even in the absence of post-traumatic arthritis, the ankle may be stiff and painful in the long term. The patient should be warned accordingly. Ankle arthrodesis may be required in the future.

## 10.6 Ankle sprains

Ankle sprains are ligament injuries and are one of the commonest sports-related injuries seen in the emergency department. Most involve the lateral ligament complex, comprising the anterior talofibular ligament, the calcaneofibular ligament and the posterior talofibular ligament (**Figure 10.1**). Other injuries, for example deltoid ligament injuries, are much less frequent (**Figure 10.2**).

### Epidemiology
Ankle ligamentous injuries are more common in men than women.

### Causes
The most common cause is inversion of the foot. However, damage can also be caused by eversion or external rotation of the foot. Ankle sprains are common in all sports.

### Clinical features
Patients present with:
- pain
- swelling
- bruising
- ligamentous tenderness
- restriction of range of motion

Patients normally have pain on weight-bearing. Traditionally, these injuries have been categorised as grade I, II and III, depending on the severity of soft tissue injury, bleeding and functional impairment (**Table 10.3**).

| Grade | Description |
|-------|-------------|
| I | Mild damage to ligament(s), no joint instability |
| II | Partial tear to ligament(s), joint becomes loose |
| III | Complete tear of ligament(s), instability of joint |

Table 10.3 Grading of ligamentous injuries of the ankle.

### Investigations

The decision whether or not to obtain radiographs of the ankle after clinical examination depends on whether the injury fulfils any of the criteria described by the Ottawa ankle rules (see Figure 10.10). If there is chronic instability or pain, MRI is used to visualise the ligamentous injury and any problems with cartilage within the ankle joint (**Figure 10.15**).

### Management

Acute ankle sprains are managed conservatively. If patients go on to have chronic symptoms, including pain and instability, then these should be investigated and managed appropriately. Surgical intervention is sometimes required.

**Conservative management** The RICE principles, i.e. rest, ice pack use, compression and elevation, are advised. The use of strapping or braces is not advised, because immobilisation usually leads to joint stiffness. Early active mobilisation (i.e. after 1–2 days of rest) with physiotherapy improves functional outcome.

**Surgical management** It is considered in patients with:
- chronic instability
- residual pain

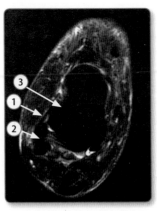

**Figure 10.15** Axial MRI showing the anterior talofibular ligament ① running between the distal and anterior aspect of the fibula ② and the talus ③.

- recurrent sprains
- an inability to return to sporting activities

Before surgical management is considered, all patients require a full rehabilitation programme. This includes ankle-strengthening exercises.

# 10.7 Talus fractures

The talus bridges the ankle joint and the joints of the midfoot (**Figures 10.1–10.3**). Talus injuries therefore affect one or more of these joints and disrupt multiple planes of movement. There is a spectrum of injuries to the talus. The ankle and subtalar joint are commonly involved.

Much of the talus is covered by articular cartilage. The blood supply is derived from two arteries: the dominant supply is from the posterior tibial artery via the artery of the tarsal canal and the deltoid branch. The remainder of the blood supply is from the anterior tibial artery and the perforating peroneal artery, via the artery of the sinus tarsi. As most of the talus has a retrograde blood supply, there is a risk of avascular necrosis with displaced fractures to the body or neck of the talus.

## Epidemiology

Talus fractures are the most common tarsal fracture after calcaneal fractures. They account for > 50% of tarsal fractures.

## Causes

Most are due to high-energy forced dorsiflexion with axial loading.

## Clinical features

The foot is swollen, tender, bruised and blistered. Because talus fractures are high-energy injuries, other musculoskeletal injuries, especially of the ipsilateral lower limb, should be sought. Compartment syndrome should be ruled out (see page 349).

## Investigations

Anteroposterior and lateral radiographs are required. CT scans are used to plan surgical intervention and assess for:

- articular involvement
- displacement
- degree of comminution
- other foot fractures

## Management

The Hawkins classification is commonly used to grade fractures of the talar neck (**Table 10.4** and **Figure 10.17**). Any dislocation of the subtalar or ankle joint associated with a talus fracture is an emergency (**Figure 10.16**); reduction must be carried out as soon as possible in either the emergency department or, more likely, in theatre.

**Conservative management** This is used only for non-displaced fractures, i.e. Hawkins type I fractures. A below-knee back slab is applied; this is converted to a full plaster of Paris cast or boot in fracture clinic. The ankle remains immobilised for 8–12 weeks and non–weight-bearing for at least 6 weeks.

**Surgical management** If the dislocation is reduced in the emergency department, definitive fixation is usually carried out the next day or when the soft tissue swelling has settled. If open reduction of the dislocation has been carried out as an emergency procedure, the fracture may not have been fixed at the same time. In such cases, definitive fixation is planned in a similar time frame when the swelling settled.

| Type | Description | Risk of avascular necrosis (%) |
|------|-------------|--------------------------------|
| I | Non-displaced | < 20 |
| II | Subtalar dislocation | 20–50 |
| III | Subtalar and tibiotalar dislocation | 20–100 |
| IV | Subtalar, tibiotalar and talonavicular dislocation | 70–100 |

Table 10.4 Hawkins classification of talus fractures

Patients remain non–weight-bearing for 8–12 weeks after the operation.

**Complications**  Patients are followed up in clinic, and regular radiographs are obtained to look for signs of avascular necrosis. Hawkins' sign (**Figure 10.17**) confirms subchondral osteopenia and usually excludes avascular necrosis. If avascular necrosis

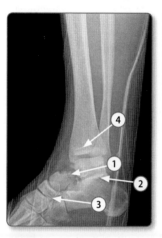

**Figure 10.16** Lateral radiograph of the ankle and hindfoot showing a Hawkins type III fracture of the talar neck ① with dislocation of the subtalar joint ②. There is significant displacement of the fracture; on this radiograph, the foot distal to the fracture ③ appears as expected on a lateral view but the ankle ④ is almost in an anteroposterior plane.

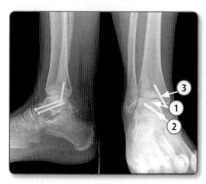

**Figure 10.17** Lateral and anteroposterior radiographs of the ankle showing a lucent line ① in the subchondral bone in the body of the talus; this is known as Hawkins' sign. Open reduction and internal fixation of the talus fracture is evident, with two screws ② across the fracture site. To gain access to fix the fracture, a medial malleolar osteotomy has been carried out and fixed with one screw ③.

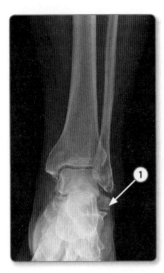

**Figure 10.18** Anteroposterior radiograph of the ankle. ① Fracture of the lateral process of the talus.

occurs, arthritis of both the ankle and subtalar joints is likely, along with collapse of the bone and significant morbidity.

Avascular necrosis may occur up to 18 months after the initial injury. Therefore patients with talar fractures are followed up for at least this length of time to ensure that avascular necrosis is not occurring.

## 10.8 Calcaneal fractures

The calcaneus is the largest tarsal bone. Through it, most of a person's body weight is transmitted from the talus to the ground.

Calcaneal fractures are the most common type of tarsal fracture. They are associated with vertebral injuries in about 10% of patients, and contralateral calcaneal injuries in 10–20%. Most calcaneal fractures are intra-articular.

## Epidemiology

Calcaneal fractures occur most commonly in those aged 18–50 years. Up to 20% of theses fractures are open injuries.

## Causes

The mechanism of injury is usually high-energy axial loading from falls or jumps from a height or motor vehicle accidents.

## Clinical features

Patients present with:
- pain in the heel
- limp
- inability to weight-bear

The foot is tender on palpation of the heel or if the heel is squeezed. The heel can look misshapen, out of alignment or flattened. The hindfoot is bruised. Patients occasionally have a haematoma extending to the sole of the foot (Mondor's sign); this is pathognomonic for calcaneal fractures.

Because calcaneal fractures are often caused by falls from a height, 10% are associated with a spinal fracture. Patients are assessed for evidence of compartment syndrome (see page 349).

## Investigations

Anteroposterior, lateral and oblique radiographs are required. On the lateral radiograph, Böhler's angle (**Figure 10.19**) and Gissane's angle are assessed. CT scans are used to define the fracture pattern and the extent of damage to the subtalar joint (**Figure 10.20**).

## Management

Calcaneal fractures are categorised as extra-articular or intra-articular. Most (>70%) are intra-articular. This classification often helps determine management. Intra-articular fractures are more prone to arthrosis in the long term.

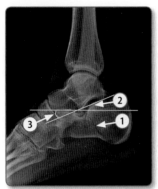

**Figure 10.19** Lateral radiograph of the ankle, showing a calcaneal fracture ①. The posterior facet of the subtalar joint ② has been rotated and flattened as a consequence of the fracture. Böhler's angle ③ has been diminished. Böhler's angle is measured at the intersection of two lines: the first drawn between the posterior superior aspect of the calcaneal tuberosity to the highest point of the posterior articular facet, and the second drawn to the anterior process of the calcaneous.

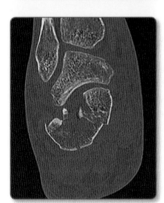

**Figure 10.20** Coronal CT of the ankle and hindfoot showing a comminuted intra-articular fracture of the calcaneum.

Calcaneal fractures, whether treated conservatively or surgically, are usually severely disabling injuries. Patients are often non–weight-bearing for up to 12 weeks. Restoration of the shape of the calcaneus, along with the articular surface of the subtalar joint, is thought to improve outcomes.

**Conservative management** This is indicated for:

- non-displaced or minimally displaced extra-articular fractures
- non-displaced intra-articular fractures

It is also considered in patients with severe injuries and who are smokers or have diabetes or peripheral vascular disease.

Initial management is a soft, padded dressing or back slab, which is applied for comfort, then as the swelling reduces, the foot is placed into a walker boot which can be removed occasionally to allow ankle movement and thereby prevent stiffness. Patients remain non–weight-bearing for up to 3 months.

**Surgical management** For displaced intra-articular and comminuted fractures, surgery is considered only after the initial swelling has subsided (up to 2 weeks after initial injury). The fractures are fixed through a large incision laterally, with a combination of a plate specific to the shape of the calcaneus and screws.

**Complications** Calcaneal fractures are at very high risk of:
- post-traumatic arthritis (subtalar or calcaneocuboid)
- stiffness
- complex regional pain syndrome
- chronic pain

Patients may never return to their former employment.

---

# 10.9 Achilles tendon ruptures

The Achilles tendon is the thickest and strongest tendon in the body. It is the convergence of the tendons of gastrocnemius and soleus, and attaches to the calcaneus. Acute rupture of the Achilles tendon usually occurs 4–6 cm above the calcaneal insertion point in its mid-substance.

Patients describe feeling or hearing a snap in the back of the ankle, or a sensation of being kicked or struck on the back of the leg. The diagnosis of an Achilles tendon rupture remains largely clinical.

## Epidemiology

Achilles tendon ruptures are most common in middle age, especially in men aged 30–50 years.

## Causes

The mechanism of injury is usually a sudden movement

involving pushing off, acceleration or change in direction. Other mechanisms include:
- an increase in the level of activity
- introduction of a new activity
- direct trauma to the tendon

The risk of rupture is increased by:
- recent local steroid injection
- systemic steroid or quinolone antibiotic injections
- previous rupture

### Clinical features

Patients have pain with a limp. However, they remain able to plantar flex the ankle because of preservation of the deep flexors.

Examination is carried out with the patient lying prone on the examination table with their feet extending over the edge (see **Figure 10.9**).
- Compare both legs and ankles
- Look for swelling and bruising
- Assess the contour of the Achilles tendon and the shape of the calves
- Look for the resting posture of both ankles on the ruptured side the ankle will be more dorsiflexed.
- Palpate for a gap in the tendon and tenderness
- Feel for tendon continuity
- Perform the calf squeeze test on both legs: if the Achilles tendon is not ruptured, the foot plantar flexes. With a rupture, the foot does not move.

### Investigations

Anteroposterior and lateral radiographs of the ankle are obtained to exclude bony injury. Ultrasound confirms the diagnosis if there is clinical ambiguity after examination. A true partial rupture is very rare, so caution is exercised when making a decision to treat based on this diagnosis.

### Management

Operative management can reduce the incidence of rerupture very slightly, although it involves the risk of complications associated with surgery. Ruptures are usually treated non-operatively if diagnosed and appropriately treated within the first 72 hours.

The aim of treatment is to maintain the length of the tendon and allow it to heal in continuity. Initially, the foot must be placed in an equinus back slab. The patient may be admitted on the day of presentation with a view to operate the following day, or referred to fracture clinic and sent home with appropriate immobilisation and crutches.

**Conservative management** The aim is to allow healing of the tendon by holding the foot in plantar flexion or ankle equinus, thus bringing the tendon ends closer together. It is indicated when:
- the patient presents within 48 h of injury
- there is no gapping of the tendon
- surgery is deemed unsuitable, for example because the patient is at high risk of anaesthetic complications or poor wound healing

Disadvantages of conservative management include the potential for an elongated tendon, leading to reduced plantar flexion power, and scar tissue forming within the gap in the tendon ends, which increases the risk of rerupture by 10 times.

**Surgical management** This allows for accurate apposition of the tendon ends and is generally considered best for active individuals. The procedure is either open or minimally invasive, depending on the surgeon's preference.

## Clinical insight

An Achilles tendon rupture identified 6 weeks after injury is considered delayed or missed. The signs are less obvious, because the gap will already have become filled with scar tissue. The calf squeeze test is unreliable at this point. Patients often complain of fatigue in the affected leg. MRI is often required to help with diagnosis.

Results of surgery for a delayed rupture are not as good as those for primary repair. Surgery may include reconstructive techniques such as tendon transfer.

## 10.10 Lisfranc (tarsometatarsal) injuries

The Lisfranc ligament connects the 2nd metatarsal base to the medial cuneiform. Lisfranc injuries are a spectrum of injuries characterised by ligamentous instability and dislocation, with or without an associated fracture, to the tarsometatarsal joints of the midfoot. It may be considered a significant ligamentous disruption.

Undiagnosed, under-treated and/or untreated Lisfranc injuries lead to high levels of morbidity and midfoot arthritis. Injuries can be subtle and therefore difficult to see on radiography.

### Epidemiology

Lisfranc injuries affect 1 in 55,000 people annually. They are more common in men and athletes, and occur at any age.

### Causes

The mechanism is usually high energy, either:
- direct, from a crush injury (e.g. being run over by a car or falling from a height), or
- indirect, from sudden rotational force on a plantar-flexed foot

### Clinical features

Lisfranc injuries are frequently very painful, with significant swelling.

A Lisfranc injury is considered in patients with midfoot pain, especially on weight-bearing, or with polytrauma injuries. Other features of this type of injury include:
- plantar ecchymosis
- deformity
- tenderness in the tarsometatarsal joints on palpation
- instability

### Investigations

An anteroposterior radiograph normally shows alignment of the medial border of the 2nd metatarsal base and the middle cuneiform (**Figure 10.21**). On an oblique radiograph, the medial border of the 4th metatarsal normally aligns with the medial

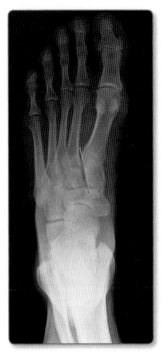

**Figure 10.21** In a standard anteroposterior radiograph of the foot, the medial side of the middle cuneiform and the medial border of the 2nd metatarsal are aligned, as indicated by the line.

border of the cuboid (**Figure 10.22**). A gap of > 2 mm between the base of the 1st and 2nd metatarsals indicates a Lisfranc injury (**Figure 10.23**).

If the injury is subtle, a weight-bearing anteroposterior radiograph may show diastasis or widening at the tarsometatarsal joints. A CT scan is mandatory if there is any doubt as to the diagnosis. When the diagnosis has been established, CT is used to define the extent of injury and guide surgical planning.

## Management

The vast majority of these injuries are managed surgically.

**Conservative management** This is suitable for completely non-displaced, stable injuries, which may have an associated fracture. A non–weight-bearing below-knee cast is worn for

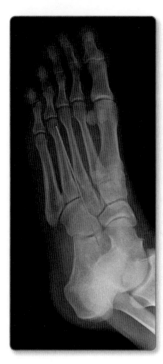

**Figure 10.22** In an oblique radiograph of the foot, the medial border of the 4th metatarsal aligns with the medial border of the cuboid.

6–8 weeks before weight-bearing and mobilisation are considered.

**Surgical management**  Most Lisfranc injuries require surgery. The gold standard is open reduction and fixation of the joints and fractures with screws and/or plates. The patient is kept non–weight-bearing for at least 6 weeks. The metalwork is usually removed after 6–9 months.

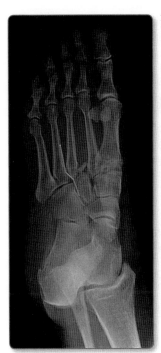

**Figure 10.23** Oblique radiograph of the foot showing a Lisfranc fracture dislocation. There is disruption of the normal architecture of the tarsometatarsal joints. There is also widening between the 2nd and 3rd metatarsals, with loss of the normal relation between the 4th metatarsal and the cuneiform.

## 10.11 Metatarsal fractures

The metatarsals provide the main weight-bearing surface during normal gait. The cascade of metatarsals has varying degrees of mobility at the tarsometatarsal joints, particularly in the sagittal plane, allowing the forefoot to accommodate walking on uneven ground.

Fractures of the metatarsals, especially if displaced, can disrupt this anatomy. Without appropriate treatment, this can lead to many long-term problems.

## Epidemiology

Metatarsal fractures are the commonest fractures of the forefoot. They are normally divided into three groups:

- 1st metatarsal fractures
- 5th metatarsal fractures (the most common)
- fractures of the 2nd, 3rd and 4th metatarsals

Fractures of the 1st and 5th metatarsals are usually seen in isolation, whereas fractures of the other metatarsals often occur multiply.

Stress fractures (also known as march fractures, as they were often found in soldiers due to the stress of marching) affect many healthy, active patients, as well as those with neuropathic conditions, rheumatoid arthritis or bone disease.

### Clinical insight

Jones fractures occur as an acute injury of fatigue fracture rather than avulsion injury. The fracture is sited in the diaphysis, within 1.5 cm of the tuberosity and lies distal to both the tarsometatarsal joint and the joint between the 4th and 5th metatarsals.

Non-union is common and surgical fixation, with or without bone grafting, may be required. Initial treatment is use of a non–weight-bearing cast for up to 6 weeks.

### Causes

Fractures of one or more metatarsals occurs as a result of an acute injury or repeated stress or overuse (**Table 10.5**).

| Mechanism | Fracture pattern |
|---|---|
| Forced inversion or eversion of forefoot | Spiral fracture |
| Crush injury | Multiple fractures and soft tissue injury |
| Sudden forced inversion | Fracture of 5th metatarsal base |
| Forced adduction or inversion with ankle plantar flexed | Jones fracture: a fracture at the metadiaphyseal junction |
| Fatigue or overuse | Stress fracture (also known as march fracture), usually of the 2nd metatarsal |

**Table 10.5** Mechanisms of injury leading to metatarsal fractures.

## Clinical features

Patients present with:

- pain
- swelling
- tenderness over the fracture site
- difficulty or inability to weight-bear because of pain

If more than one metatarsal is fractured, this can lead to gross swelling and deformity.

The patient must be assessed carefully for any evidence of compartment syndrome. Lisfranc injury is considered and open

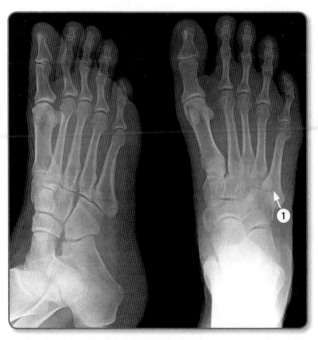

**Figure 10.24** Anteroposterior and oblique radiographs of the foot showing an avulsion fracture to the base of the 5th metatarsal.

injuries sought; these require appropriate wound management. On palpation, there is usually tenderness over the fracture site. There may be obvious instability. The range of motion of forefoot and toes are compared with that in the uninjured foot. Pulses and sensation are checked.

## Investigations

Anteroposterior, lateral and oblique radiographs of the foot are required. The metatarsophalangeal joints are examined carefully for signs of dislocation. Fractures are described by:

- metatarsal number
- location
- type
- displacement
- articular involvement

Stress fractures may not be apparent at first presentation; MRI may be needed to confirm the diagnosis. A stress fracture that has been present for some time usually with callus visible on the radiograph. CT can be used for further imaging of multiple fractures or to rule out Lisfranc injuries. MRI is also used to identify stress fractures.

### Clinical insight

Accessory bones at the lateral aspect of the foot and may look like a fracture. Interpret in the light of the clinical findings: if there is no bony tenderness, a fracture is unlikely (**Figure 10.25**).

### Clinical insight

Be aware that in children the epiphysis at the 5th metatarsal base can be mistaken for a fracture, but also that fracture and separation at the epiphysis may occur. Consider the findings on clinical examination.

## Management

Most metatarsal shaft fractures are stable and are generally treated non-operatively. Fractures of the 5th metatarsal occur as distinct entities, including the Jones fracture. Unstable displaced metatarsal neck or head fractures require reduction and fixation.

Patients with significant soft tissue swelling require admission to hospital for rest and elevation. They are at risk

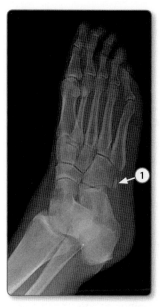

**Figure 10.25** Oblique radiograph of the foot showing the os peroneum ①. Note the smooth rounded borders and typical position, adjacent to the cuboid on the oblique view.

of developing compartment syndrome, especially in the case of crush injuries.

**Conservative management** Most isolated fractures are managed conservatively, either in plaster or a walker boot.

> ## Clinical insight
>
> Ottawa foot rules (see page 280): order foot radiographs only if the patient has pain and an inability to weight-bear for four steps, or has any bony tenderness at the navicular or base of the 5th metatarsal.

Non-union is common in Jones fractures, so these need to be identified.

**Surgical management** Fractures involving the articular surface of the 1st metatarsal head require operative treatment to ensure restoration of normal anatomy and prevent arthrosis later. Metatarsal fractures are fixed with small plates and screws. Kirschner wires are sometimes used. Operative fixation may be considered initially for athletes with a Jones fracture.

**Complications**  Common complications include:
- post-traumatic arthritis (of the tarsometatarsal and meta-tarsophalangeal joints)
- metatarsalgia
- chronic pain
- gait problems

# 10.12 Phalangeal fractures

Toes are vulnerable to injury because of their position; they are prone to being stubbed, stepped on, or having items fall on them. Fractures, dislocations and nail injuries should all be considered.

Fractures can occur at the proximal, middle or distal (terminal) phalanx. The great toe (hallux) has only two phalanges: proximal and distal. Stress fractures occur in the toes, typically in the proximal phalanx. Not all fractures of the foot phalanges require orthopaedic referral.

## Epidemiology

Phalangeal fractures are very common as a result of trauma, particularly that sustained when the patient was barefoot or not wearing protective footwear. The incidence is not clearly defined, because many people will not seek treatment.

## Causes

The mechanism of injury is usually direct trauma. Proximal phalangeal fractures are more likely with a stubbing-type injury, whereas distal or terminal phalangeal fractures usually result from crushing injuries such as a heavy weight falling on an unprotected foot.

## Clinical features

Patients present with:
- pain, including painful weight-bearing
- swelling
- bruising

There may be an obvious deformity in cases of displaced fracture or dislocation. The toes are assessed for rotational or angulated deformity. The patient's sensation and capillary refill time are checked.

Patients less commonly present with:

- subungual haematoma
- separation of the nail from the nail bed
- open wounds
- tenderness on palpation
- reduced and painful range of motion

## Investigations

Anteroposterior, lateral and oblique radiographs of the toes enable identification of the fracture and help with recognition of any fracture displacement. Any intra-articular involvement of the fracture, which increases the risk of arthritis, is noted. Signs of a dislocated joint are sought.

## Management

The majority of phalangeal fractures will be treated conservatively.

**Conservative management** Most phalangeal fractures are stable and are treated by neighbour strapping, using adhesive tape to support the fractured toe against the adjacent toe for 2–4 weeks. Patients can weight-bear as tolerated, but if the great toe is fractured a walking plaster with toe platform is usually more comfortable.

Closed, non-displaced fractures are unlikely to require orthopaedic review. Displaced fractures or dislocated toes are reduced by traction and splinted.

Open wounds are cleaned and the wound edges approximated. Subungual haematomas require decompressing by trephining; a hot sterile needle or electrocautery are used.

**Surgical management** For open fractures, surgical management comprises irrigation and debridement followed by closure of the wound. Antibiotics are prescribed to reduce the risk of osteomyelitis. The nail is retained if it can be salvaged. Open reduction and internal rotation is considered for displaced intra-articular fractures of the hallux.

**Complications** Common complications include:

- malunion or non-union
- infection
- osteomyelitis
- nail bed deformity

## 10.13 Other conditions

### Navicular fractures

Navicular fractures are an uncommon midfoot fracture (**Figure 10.26**). The navicular bone transfers forces from the hindfoot to the forefoot. Consider a navicular stress fracture in any young athlete presenting with midfoot pain.

Patients present with pain in the midfoot. Radiographs are usually sufficient to make a diagnosis. If there is uncertainty

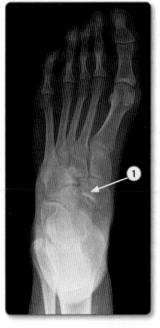

**Figure 10.26** Anteroposterior radiograph of the foot, showing a navicular fracture ①.

and a bony injury is suspected, CT is needed to confirm a fracture.

Non-displaced or minimally displaced fractures are managed with use of a below-knee cast for 4–6 weeks. Displaced fractures are treated operatively with open reduction and internal fixation, with or without bone graft. If there is extensive comminution, a primary arthrodesis is considered. Non-union, malunion, osteonecrosis and arthritis are all common complications of both displaced and non-displaced fractures.

## Plantar fasciitis

Plantar fasciitis is a painful condition of the plantar fascia, a ligamentous structure that runs across the bottom of the foot. It has previously been described as common in long-distance runners, police officers and other workers who are required to walk and stand for long periods, and is associated with obesity. It is usually caused by subtle loss of the medial arch of the foot.

Patients complain of a stabbing pain on the plantar surface of the foot, particularly the heel. This is especially apparent as they start walking in the morning or with their first few steps (start-up pain). The diagnosis is clinical. Management includes rest, physiotherapy, use of orthotics or night splints and anti-inflammatory medications.

## Foreign body in foot

If the foreign body is obvious, visible and in a safe region, it can be removed in the emergency department once the patient has been given local anaesthetic. If not, a radiograph can be obtained to help locate the foreign body, thereby enabling its removal. Patients may need surgery to fully explore the wound.

There are anatomical, biochemical and biomechanical differences between child and adult bones, as listed in **Table 11.1**. The principles of paediatric orthopaedic treatment are:

- Union is almost always possible
- Children's bones have great capacity for remodelling
- Malrotation is unacceptable at any age
- The limits of bone remodeling define the 'limits of acceptability'

Remodelling ability depends on age, location and plane of fracture, degree of deformity and the movement of adjacent joints.

## 11.1 Clinical scenario

### Child with a limp

#### Background

A 5-year-old boy presents to the emergency department with a limp. His mother says that he was fine yesterday, but that he started complaining of pain in his hip last night and has avoided putting any weight on his right leg since waking this morning. He is normally fit and well but had a cough and sore

| Anatomical | Presence of growth plate |
|---|---|
| | Thick, vascular periosteum |
| | Cambium layer has increased osteoblastic activity. |
| Biochemical | More collagen per unit area of mineralised bone |
| | Collagen is mainly type 1 |
| Biomechanical | Bone is more porous |
| | The bone has lower modulus of elasticity |
| | Lesser bending strength required to produce deformity. |

**Table 11.1** Differences of children's bones compared to adult bones.

throat last week. As far as she knows, he has had no falls or any other injuries.

## History

The patient has no notable past medical or drug history. He lives with his parents and older sister. His vaccinations are up to date. He was born at term via normal vaginal delivery.

## Examination

The boy is refusing to walk on his right leg, and is holding the right hip flexed. No bony tenderness is present. Regarding active movement, he is refusing to move the leg or hip. Passively, the hip can be flexed to 90°, but there is pain on internal and external rotation, abduction and adduction. He is apyrexial and appears well.

## Differential diagnosis

Paediatric hip pain has several differential diagnoses:
- septic arthritis
- transient synovitis or irritable hip
- Perthes' disease (Legg–Calvé–Perthes disease)
- slipped upper femoral epiphysis
- fracture
- soft tissue injury
- knee injury
- testicular pain

The most important diagnosis to exclude is septic arthritis. However, given the preceding history of a viral illness coupled with the hip being passively flexed to 90°, transient synovitis is more likely.

## Investigations

Radiographs, including an anteroposterior pelvic radiograph and frog-leg views, are obtained. These show no specific abnormailty. Blood tests include full blood count, erythrocyte sedimentation rate and C-reactive protein. US of the hip shows a small effusion. Inflammatory markers and the white cell count are normal.

The clinical picture, normal radiographs and inflammatory markers, make transient synovitis the most likely diagnosis. The small hip effusion is in keeping with this diagnosis. The patient is admitted to hospital overnight for strict rest, observation and analgesia.

## 11.2 Examination

When examining children, especially young children, involve their parents, toys and play therapists in order to get as much co-operation from the child as possible. Observe how they move, play and interact with others when relaxed. It is not as easy to stick to a strict 'look, feel, move' structure of assessment, but ensure all these aspects are still covered.

Non-accidental injury should always be considered: perform a full examination to look for bruising, skin marks and any other sites of injury away from the presenting problem.

## 11.3 Growth plate fractures

Children and young adults are at risk of growth plate injuries. Growth plates (physes) are areas of developing cartilage near the ends of long bones; they are the last parts of the bone to ossify.

**Figure 11.1** shows the anatomy of the growth plate, and its different layers. The growth plate is weaker than the rest of the bone, ligaments and muscles, and therefore vulnerable to injury.

Growth plate fractures must be recognised, because failure to do so can lead to premature fusion of the growth plate. This results in limb shortening or unequal growth, leading to deformity and disability.

### Epidemiology

About 20% of all childhood fractures are fractures of the growth plate. These occur twice as frequently in boys than girls. The fracture is most commonly at the wrist, ankle or fingers, but any of the long bones can be affected.

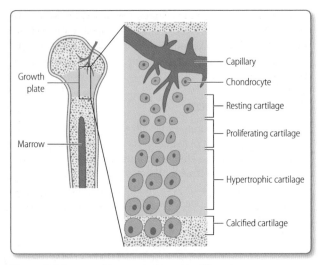

**Figure 11.1** Anatomy of the growth plate and its different layers.

## Causes

This type of fracture is most commonly caused by trauma, for example from a fall from a climbing frame or an injury sustained while playing a competitive sport. It sometimes results from chronic overuse, for example in gymnasts and long-distance runners.

## Clinical features

The patient typically presents with pain, swelling, deformity and inability to move the injured bone. The entire extremity must be assessed, because children may be unable to localise the injury. Neurovascular examination is carried out and the findings documented.

## Investigations

Anteroposterior and lateral radiographs are obtained, both of the bone and the joint above and below it. If there is uncertainty about the site of injury, radiographs of the whole limb are required.

Growth plate injuries are categorised using the Salter–Harris classification; this links radiographic appearance to clinical outcome (**Table 11.2** and **Figure 11.2**). Salter–Harris type I injuries have a good prognosis, but type V injuries have a poor prognosis. CT is sometimes required to assess the fracture pattern. **Figure 11.3** shows a Salter–Harris type II fracture of the distal tibia.

## Management

The goal of management is to accurately reduce the growth plate, restoring normal anatomy. The fracture is held with a combination of plaster of Paris cast, K wires, screws and flexible intramedullary nails. Accurate reduction has a good prognosis, but even with perfect reduction and fixation premature growth

| Type | Frequency (%) | Prognosis for normal growth |
|------|---------------|------------------------------|
| I    | < 10          | Satisfactory                 |
| II   | 70            | Satisfactory                 |
| III  | 5–10          | Satisfactory                 |
| IV   | 10            | Guarded                      |
| V    | 1             | Poor                         |

**Table 11.2** Salter–Harris classification fractures involving the growth plate.

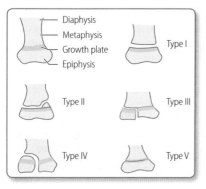

**Figure 11.2** The Salter-Harris classification of growth plate injuries.

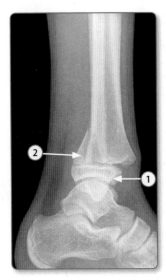

**Figure 11.3** Lateral radiograph showing a Salter–Harris type II fracture of the distal tibia. The epiphysis and physis ① have separated from the metaphysis. The small metaphyseal triangular fragment (Thurstan Holland fragment) ② is typical of this injury.

arrest cannot be guaranteed. In general, physeal fractures are difficult to manipulate after 2 weeks.

**Conservative management**  For most Salter–Harris type I immobilisation in a back slab is sufficient initially. After 1 week, when the swelling has reduced, this is converted to a full plaster or fibreglass cast. Most Salter–Harris II fractures require manipulation under anaesthetic with or without K wire fixation.

**Surgical management**  Salter–Harris type III and IV fractures require anatomical reduction; this can be done by manipulation under anaesthesia and plaster application under image intensifier guidance, manipulation under anaesthesia with percutaneous fixation or K wiring, or open reduction and internal fixation. Growth plate fractures need to be followed up for at least a year to ensure good long-term outcomes; the fracture must be assessed to detect any growth arrest or asymmetrical growth and to check that no further surgery is required.

**Complications**  Potential complications are:
- growth arrest and limb length discrepancy
- limb deformity
- avascular necrosis

## 11.4 Supracondylar humeral fractures

These are fractures in the distal third of the humerus, just proximal to the trochlea and capitellum. The fracture pattern is usually transverse.

### Epidemiology

Supracondylar humeral fractures are most common in 5- to 8-year olds. Boys are more frequently affected.

### Causes

These fractures are usually the consequence of a fall on to outstretched extended arm; this mechanism of injury produces the more common extension type of supra-condylar humeral fracture (> 95%). Flexion type injuries are normally the result of falls on to flexed elbows.

### Clinical features

Children present with a swollen, painful elbow that they are reluctant to move. They occasionally also have a clinical deformity. A thorough neurovascular examination is carried out to assess the median, radial and ulnar nerves, the distal pulses and capillary refill. The results must be clearly documented before and after any intervention.

> **Clinical insight**
>
> The brachial artery may be injured in cases of displaced fracture. If the radial pulse is absent, the temperature, colour and neurological status of the limb needs to be evaluated and the results documented. A vascular surgeon is contacted if there are any concerns. Failure to identify an arterial injury may result in Volkmann's ischaemic contracture.

> **Clinical insight**
>
> The position of the capitellum in relation to the anterior humeral line is a key finding in the assessment of elbow radiographs in children. Usually a third or more of the capitellum lies anterior to this line (**Figure 11.4**). If it does not, then a supracondylar fracture is likely (**Figure 11.5**).

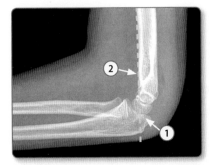

**Figure 11.4** Lateral radiograph of the elbow. Normally, at least a third of the capitellum ① is anterior to the anterior humeral line ②.

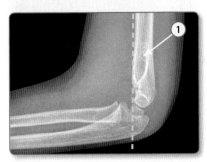

**Figure 11.5** Lateral radiograph of a type 2 supracondylar fracture. Most of the capitellum lies posterior to the anterior humeral line ①. This finding strongly suggests a fracture.

## Investigations

Anteroposterior and lateral radiographs of the elbow are obtained. CT angiography is required if there is vascular concern but the hand is pink and warm.

## Management

The Gartland classification is used to categorise extension supracondylar humeral fractures by degree of displacement (**Table 11.3** and **Figure 11.6**). Management is guided by whether the injury is a Gartland type I, II or III fracture.

Type I fractures require immobilisation in an above-elbow back slab at about 90° flexion. When the swelling has reduced, the back slab is converted to a full cast, which is worn for 3–4 weeks.

| Type | Degree of displacement |
|------|------------------------|
| I | Non-displaced |
| II | Displaced with intact posterior cortex; may be angulated or rotated |
| III | Complete displacement |

**Table 11.3** Gartland classification of supracondylar humeral fractures.

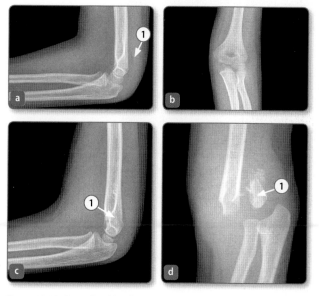

**Figure 11.6** Radiographs of the elbow, showing supracondylar humeral fractures. (a) Lateral view showing a Gartland type 1 fracture. No displacement or angulation of this fracture is evident on this view; the clue to the nature of the injury is the posterior fat pad sign ①. A posterior fat pad is almost always associated with an elbow fracture, which may be occult. The fat pad is usually raised off the posterior aspect of the numerus by a haemarthrosis. (b) anteroposterior view showing a Gartland type II fracture. (c) Lateral view showing a Gartland type II fracture. The posterior cortex is intact, but the fracture line ① is visible and has opened the anterior cortex causing the distal humerus to angulate posteriorly. (d) Lateral view showing a Gartland type III fracture. The distal humeral fracture fragment ① is completely 'off-ended' (complete loss of contact between the two fracture fragments).

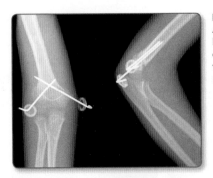

**Figure 11.7**
Anteroposterior (left) and lateral elbow radiographs demostrating Kirschner wires used to maintain reduction.

Type II fractures require manipulation under anaesthesia and application of an above-elbow plaster. If the fracture is unstable, percutaneous fixation with Kirschner wires is required to hold the position.

Type III fractures all need some form of fixation after manipulation under anaesthesia. Fixation is by either percutaneous Kirschner wire fixation, or in cases of severe displacement and comminution or failure of closed reduction, open reduction and internal fixation with stabilisation of the fracture by Kirschner wires (**Figure 11.7**).

**Complications** Common complications of supracondylar humeral fractures are:
- injury to the brachial artery
- loss of full elbow extension
- deformity
- injury to the median or anterior interosseous nerve
- ulnar nerve injury (often iatrogenic)
- radial nerve injury
- compartment syndrome

## 11.5 Condylar fractures

Condylar fractures make up around 20% of paediatric elbow fractures. The lateral condyle is more commonly injured than the medial, although both can be caused by a fall on to an outstretched hand.

The most common condylar injury to the medial side is the medial epicondylar fracture, which is caused by an avulsion secondary to a valgus stress at the elbow. Up to 50% of these fracture are associated with elbow dislocation. Failure to diagnose and manage condylar fractures comes with a high risk of deformity. It is essential to ensure that the epicondyle is not trapped within the joint: missed or late presentations of condylar fractures lead to malunion and deformity, with impaired elbow function and reduced range of movement.

> **Clinical insight**
>
> Key points to remember when assessing radiographs of the elbow are:
> - a visible anterior fat pad is normal
> - displacement of the anterior fat pad suggests fracture
> - a visible posterior fat pad (**Figure 11.6a**) is always abnormal; this finding makes fracture a more likely diagnosis
> - absence of a visible fat pad does not exclude fracture

## Epidemiology

Lateral condylar fractures (**Figure 11.8**) are more common than medial condylar fractures (**Figure 11.9**). Lateral condyle fractures are most common in children aged 5–8 years; medial epicondylar fractures occur in children aged 9–14 years.

## Causes

Condylar fractures are caused by:
- direct trauma to the elbow as a consequence of a fall on to a flexed elbow

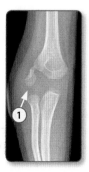

**Figure 11.8** Anteroposterior radiograph of the elbow, showing a fracture of the lateral condyle.

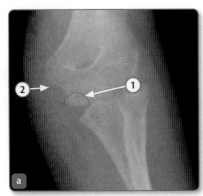

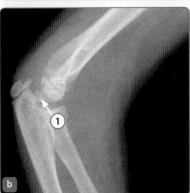

**Figure 11.9** (a) Anteroposterior elbow radiograph showing a medical condylar fracture. The medial epicondyle ① has fractured and displaced from its anatomical position ②. The fragment now sits in the elbow joint. (b) Lateral radiograph of medial epicondylar fracture the epicondyle ① now sits in the elbow joint.

- indirect trauma from a fall on to an outstretched arm, with either varus stress, resulting in fracture of the lateral condyle, or valgus stress, resulting in fracture of the medial epicondyle

## Clinical features

Diagnosis is less obvious than with supracondylar fractures, because there may be very little swelling and no deformity. The child will complain of pain at the elbow and be reluctant to move their arm. Localised bony tenderness is present on palpation and all movement of the elbow is painful.

### Investigations

Anteroposterior and lateral radiographs of the elbow are required. A CT scan is helpful if the diagnosis is uncertain. In young patients whose growth plates have not all ossified, arthrography is useful to differentiate between a fracture and normal anatomy.

### Management

The management is guided by the nature and displacement of the fracture.

**Conservative management** Non-displaced or minimally displaced fractures are treated by immobilisation in an above-elbow back slab in 90° flexion. This is converted to a full above-elbow plaster of Paris cast, which remains in place for 4–6 weeks.

> ## Guiding principle
>
> CRITOL is a mnemonic for the order of appearance of the ossification centres in the paediatric elbow (**Table 11.4** and **Figure 11.10**). It is helpful when distinguishing between a fracture, an avulsion fragment and a normal apophysis because you can tell which ossification centres are yet to close.
>
> Although, rarely, the order of ossification can vary, the trochlea always ossifies after the internal (medial) epicondyle. Therefore if the trochlea is visible, the internal (medial) epicondyle should be present; if not, it may be trapped in the joint (**Figure 11.9b** and **11.11**).

**Surgical management** Minimally displaced fractures may benefit from manipulation under anaesthesia and application of a plaster of Paris cast. For unstable, completely displaced fractures, open reduction and internal fixation is required; Kirschner wires are used to

| Ossification centre | Approximate age at appearance |
| --- | --- |
| Capitellum | 6–12 months |
| Radial head | 1–2 years |
| Internal (medial) epicondyle | 3–4 years |
| Trochlea | 5–6 years |
| Olecranon | 8–9 years |
| Lateral epicondyle | 11–12 years |

**Table 11.4** CRITOL mnemonic for the names and order of appearance of the ossification centres of the elbow.

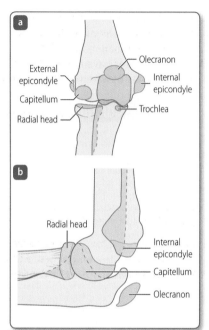

**Figure 11.10** Anatomy of paediatric elbow. (a) AP view. (b) Lateral view

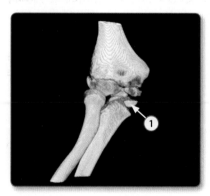

**Figure 11.11** CT reconstruction showing the medial epicondyle ① in the elbow joint. On an anteroposterior radiograph, the unexpected absence of the medial epicondyle prompts suspicion that the fragment may be in the joint.

hold the fracture fragment in place, then the elbow is placed in a cast at 90° flexion. In older children screw fixation is more desirable: as children transition into adolescence the forces acting across the elbow increase as a consequnce of an increase in mass and power. This causes fracture displacement if held only with K wires.

**Complications**  Common complications of condylar fracture are:

- deformity
- ulnar nerve injury
- avascular necrosis
- non-union

# 11.6 Radial head and neck fractures

Radial head and neck fractures account for 5% of paediatric elbow fractures. They commonly occur as a consequence of a fall onto an outstretched hand and are associated with elbow dislocation.

## Epidemiology

In children, radial neck fractures are much more common than radial head fractures, which are rare. They both most commonly present in children aged 9–10 years.

## Causes

Radial head and neck fractures are most commonly the result of falls on to an outstretched hand or chronic repetitive stress injuries, for example throwing injuries.

## Clinical features

Children present with lateral swelling of the elbow and pain, particularly on any movement of the elbow. Younger children occasionally present with referred wrist pain.

### Clinical insight

When assessing elbow radiographs, draw the radiocapitellar line. This line runs along the long axis of the proximal radius and should pass through the centre of the capitellum on the lateral radiograph. If it does not, a dislocated radial head is suspected.

### Investigations

Anteroposterior and lateral radiographs of the elbow are required (**Figure 11.12**). Oblique views may also be helpful. Comparison with radiographs of the other elbow helps identify subtle abnormalities.

MRI scans are used in children whose growth plates have not yet ossified and in whom there is doubt about whether a fracture is present.

### Management

The management of radial head and neck fractures depends on the acceptable level of angulation versus anatomical reduction. Early mobilisation is encouraged to prevent elbow stiffness.

**Conservative management** A non-displaced or minimally displaced fracture (< 30° angulation) is treated by immobilisation in a collar and cuff or cast for 1–2 weeks, followed by early range-of-motion exercises.

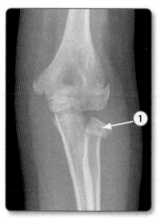

**Figure 11.12** Anteroposterior radiograph showing fracture dislocation of the radial head ①.

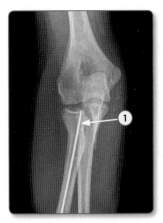

**Figure 11.13** Anteroposterior elbow radiograph showing flexible intramedullary nail fixation ① for fracture dislocation of the radial head.

**Surgical management** Fractures with 30–60° of angulation require closed manipulation under anaesthesia followed by immobilisation in an above-elbow cast in pronation and 90° of flexion for about 2 weeks. Fractures with > 60° of angulation require either closed reduction and percutaneous Kirschner wire fixation or open reduction and internal fixation with Kirschner wire fixation, depending on the stability. Flexible intermedullary nails are frequently used to manage such fractures (**Figure 11.13**).

**Complications** Common complications of radial head and neck fractures are:

- stiffness and reduced range of movement
- avascular necrosis of the radial head
- posterior interosseous nerve injury
- radioulnar synostosis
- myositis ossificans
- overgrowth of the radial head

## 11.7 Radial head subluxation

Radial head subluxation makes up 25% of paediatric elbow injuries and is also known as pulled elbow or nursemaid's elbow.

### Epidemiology
Radial head subluxation most common in girls aged 2–3 years, and is more common in the left elbow.

### Causes
The typical history is the sudden pulling of an extended forearm, for example when a parent or carer jerks a child back from the road to avoid oncoming traffic (hence why it is more common in the left elbow: because the child's carer is more likely to be holding them with their right-hand). The injury is the consequence of stretching of the annular ligament, which slips proximally on the radial head.

### Clinical features
The child or their parent or carer describes the typical history for radial head subluxation, and may even report an audible pop or snap. The child presents with pain. They hold the arm with the elbow flexed and forearm pronated, refusing to move it. Tenderness is present on palpation.

### Investigations
There are no radiographic abnormalities. The diagnosis is clinical; radiological studies are not indicated.

### Management
Closed reduction is carried out in the emergency department; the forearm is supinated and then flexed while pressure is applied over the radial head. There is likely to be a palpable click. It is extremely rare for closed reduction to fail and for open reduction with repair of the annular ligament to be necessary.

**Complications**  Common complications are:
- recurrence
- missed diagnosis

## 11.8 Hip problems: slipped upper femoral epiphysis

Slipped upper femoral epiphysis is displacement of the epiphysis in relation to the femur. The epiphysis remains inside the acetabulum while the femoral neck moves anteriorly and rotates externally. The presenting features are pain and a limp. The pain may have been on going for weeks or sometimes months. More commonly the onset is acute.

## Epidemiology

Slipped upper femoral epiphysis is more common in boys at the average age of 12 years. It is more likely to occur in children who are overweight. Over 25% of cases involve both hips.

## Causes

The greatest risk factor is obesity, but the injury is also associated with hypothyroidism and chronic renal failure.

## Clinical features

Slipped upper femoral epiphysis typically presents with pain in the hip, knee or both. It can present with isolated knee pain, which distracts from hip investigations; examine the hip as well to ensure the diagnosis is not missed. Other clinical features include pain on internal rotation, reduced hip movements, hip weakness and abnormal gait.

## Investigations

An anteroposterior and a frog-leg view of the pelvis are obtained (**Figures 11.14** and **11.15**). In cases of uncertainty, MRI is helpful.

> ## Clinical insight
>
> A hip problem is considered in any case of a child presenting with knee pain. Examination of the joint above and below the knee, i.e. the hip and ankle, is essential because many childhood hip pathologies present with knee pain alone.

## Management

Operative management is needed: either percutaneous or open surgery to carry out anatomical reduction and insert screws across the physis. The other hip is usually fixed prophylactically, because there is a risk of slipped upper femoral epiphysis on the contralateral side in up to 50% of cases (**Figure 11.16**).

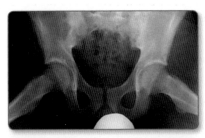

**Figure 11.14** Frog-leg lateral radiograph of the pelvis.

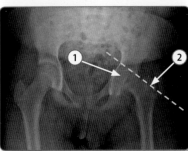

**Figure 11.15** Anteroposterior pelvic radiograph showing a slipped upper femoral epiphysis to the left side. This shows Trethowan's sign; the femoral head ① sits inferiorly to Klein's line ②, a line drawn along the lateral border of the femoral neck.

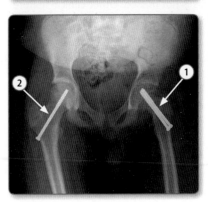

**Figure 11.16** Anteroposterior pelvic radiograph showing pinning of the slipped upper femoral epiphysis on the left side ①, with prophylactic pinning of the contralateral hip ②.

**Complications** Common complications include:

- avascular necrosis of the femoral head
- contralateral slipped upper femoral epiphysis
- leg length discrepancy
- gait disturbance
- early onset osteoarthritis

## 11.9 Hip problems: Perthes' disease

In Perthes' disease, blood flow to the femoral head is disrupted, thereby causing avascular necrosis of the femoral epiphysis. Clinically and radiologically the signs are subtle; if there is any doubt an MRI scan is used to elicit the diagnosis.

### Epidemiology

The condition occurs most commonly in children aged 4–8 years. Boys are five times more likely to be affected.

### Causes

The cause of Perthes' disease is unknown, but risk factors include obesity, family history, passive smoking (usually parental), clotting abnormalities, low socioeconomic status, male sex and previous trauma. Perthes' disease is also associated with attention deficit hyperactivity disorder.

### Clinical features

The condition usually presents with insidious onset of a limp, which can be either painful or not. If pain is present, it radiates from the groin to the knee.

Examination typically finds leg shortening or reduced range of movement and stiffness at the hip joint. Alternatively, the signs in the hip may be very subtle, such as mild restriction in internal rotation. Perthes' disease is bilateral in over 10% of cases, with the disease at a different stage in each hip.

### Investigations

Anteroposterior and frog-leg radiographs are required. The femoral head typically has an irregular appearance (**Figure 11.17**), with widening of the joint space. An MRI scan is usually carried out to confirm the diagnosis and stage the disease. A hip arthrogram is used to confirm the morphology and congruency of the hip joint.

### Management

Perthes' disease is managed operatively or non-operatively, depending on the patient's age and sex and the stage of the

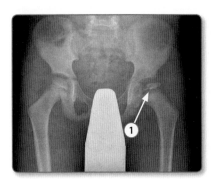

**Figure 11.17**
Anteroposterior pelvic radiograph, showing Perthes' disease at the left femoral head (1). The capital epiphysis is small, irregular and sclerotic.

disease. The longer the femoral head has to remodel once the disease has resolved the better the prognosis (hence younger patients have better outcomes). Surgery contains the femoral head to improve the chance of remodelling and congruency, achieved either by a pelvic osteotomy or osteotomy to the femoral neck.

- Non-operative treatment consists of a period of rest and use of a brace to hold the hip in abduction
- Operative management is either femoral or pelvic osteotomy

**Prognosis**  This depends on the shape of the healed femoral head and the alignment of the joint with the acetabulum. It also depends on the patient's age at presentation; the prognosis is better in children younger than 6 years. Female patients have a worse prognosis.

## 11.10 Hip problems: transient synovitis

Transient synovitis is a common cause of hip pain in children, although other joints such as the knee may be affected. The pain is caused by inflammation of the hip synovium in response to a remote bacterial or viral infection. The condition is self-limiting.

Patients sometimes present with very severe hip pain that mimics septic arthritis. If this is the case septic arthritis should be excluded before transient synovitis can be diagnosed.

## Epidemiology

Transient synovitis presents between 4 and 8 years of age, and is twice as common in boys.

## Causes

The cause of the condition is unknown, however it is thought to be related to viral or bacterial infections, either directly or via circulating toxins.

## Clinical features

Typically, the child appears well. Common features are:

- mild temperature
- hip is painful to move actively and passively with moderate restriction
- child walks with a limp or refuses to weight-bear on the affected side

There is often a history of viral infection such as a sore throat or cold in the week preceding the onset of hip symptoms.

## Investigations

Anteroposterior pelvis radiographs for both hips and a frog lateral radiograph are taken. Ultrasounds show a small effusion and synovial thickening, although they cannot distinguish between transient synovitis and septic arthritis. If septic arthritis cannot be excluded a hip aspiration is undertaken. Blood tests for inflammatory markers may be mildly raised, but are usually normal.

## Management

Rest and analgesia is usually all that is required. The symptoms are self-limiting and resolve within 48 hours of onset. There is no long-term consequence of transient synovitis.

# 11.11 Femoral shaft fractures

Fractures of the femoral shaft account for about 2% of paediatric fractures. They are more common in the summer months when more outdoor activities occur. Femoral shaft fractures are most commonly caused by falls mobile children less than 10 years old and by high-energy trauma in adolescents. If the fracture is as a result of mild trauma a pathological cause should be sought.

## Epidemiology
Femoral shaft fractures peak in incidence between the ages of 2 and 4 years and in mid-adolescence.

## Causes
In children who are yet to walk, 80% of femoral shaft fractures are the result of non-accidental injury. Over 90% of cases in older children are caused by road traffic accidents.

## Clinical features
Children with a femoral shaft fracture present with pain, swelling, deformity and inability to weight-bear. In paediatric trauma patients, a full assessment must take place; splints and bandages applied before arrival at hospital are removed to assess the soft tissue and exclude open fracture.

Trauma patients are treated in accordance with the Advanced Trauma Life Support protocol, to avoid distraction by the obvious injuries.

## Investigations
Anteroposterior and lateral radiographs are required.

## Management
Management of femoral shaft fractures depends on the patient's age and the position of the fracture (**Table 11.4**).

In children younger than 6 months, a hip spica cast is applied at the time of fracture reduction, usually under general anaesthetic. In the fixed position, the hips are flexed to 60–90° and in 30° of abduction and the knees flexed to about 90° (**Figure 11.18**). Pressure on the popliteal fossa must be avoided to prevent compression of the popliteal artery, posterior tibial nerve and peroneal nerve. Pressure sores should be monitored for. Also, the parents or carers must be able to recognise and report and neurovascular changes. They must

| Patient characteristics | Fracture characteristics | Treatment |
|---|---|---|
| 0–5 years old | With or without < 3 cm of shortening | Hip spica cast |
| 7 months to 5 years old | With > 3 cm of shortening | Traction for 2–3 weeks, then delayed hip spica cast |
| 6–10 years old and < 45 kg | – | Femoral flexible intramedullary nail (with nail removal at 1 year) |
| > 11 years old | – | ORIF with plate or flexible intermedullary nail |
| Polytrauma patient | – | External fixation |

Table 11.4 Treatment of femoral shaft fractures in children.

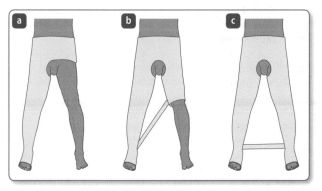

Figure 11.18 Types of hip spica. In younger children it is sometimes necessary to put both legs in plaster (c) to control the fracture. In older children a single leg spica (a) or a spica with control bar (b) is used depending on the nature of the fracture.

also be able to attend to the child's hygiene needs while the spica is in place.

In a child up to 5 years old, a femoral shaft fracture is managed in a Thomas splint. In children older than 5 years, flexible intramedullary nailing or plating of the fracture may be considered.

**Complications**  Common complications are:

- non-union or malunion
- leg length discrepancy and associated gait disturbance
- osteonecrosis of the femoral head
- repeat fracture

Because of increased blood supply to the healing fracture, a femoral shaft may lengthen by > 1 cm. Therefore, when reducing the fracture it is deliberately shortened by 1 cm.

# 11.12 Tibial fractures

Tibial fractures are divided into injuries involving the epiphysis, the metaphysis and the shaft (diaphysis). The goal of management is to prevent growth complications and deformity.

On average, the epiphyseal plate to the proximal tibia closes at 14 years of age in girls and 16 years of age in boys. Leg length increases by an average of about 23 mm per year, of which 15 mm is in the knee, so fractures resulting in growth reduction have a significant effect on gait and function.

## Epidemiology and causes

Epiphyseal fractures are rare but must be identified, because they are associated with compartment syndrome and vascular damage (the popliteal artery trifurcates posteriorly to the epiphysis). They are high-energy injuries.

Metaphyseal fractures usually occur in children aged 3–6 years. They are low-impact injuries caused by valgus force to the knee.

Tibial shaft fractures make up 15% of paediatric fractures. Up to 30% of tibial shaft fractures also involve the fibula. Most are the result of road traffic accidents or are toddler's fractures.

## Clinical features

Tibial shaft fractures present with pain, swelling, inability to weight-bear and vastly reduced range of movement. The presentation is similar regardless of the exact position of the fracture. In epiphyseal fractures, distal perfusion must be fully assessed.

## Investigations

An anteroposterior and a lateral radiograph of the knee and lower leg are required. If there is any concern about the joints above and below, radiographs of the hip and ankle are also obtained. The fibula is always also checked for fractures.

> ### Guiding principle
>
> A toddler's fracture is a non-displaced spiral fracture of the tibial shaft. It occurs in walking toddlers under 3 years old. It is caused by low-impact trauma and rotational injuries, and usually involves the distal tibia. This type of fracture takes about 3–4 weeks to heal.

## Management

**Conservative management**  Over 95% of fractures of tibial fractures  are treated non-operatively by application of a long leg cast, with the knee flexed to about 45° to minimise rotation. This is followed by a radiographic check 1–2 weeks later and review at the fracture clinic.

**Surgical management**  This consists of anatomical reduction and fixation using pins, plates or screws, or a combination of these. Many centres use flexible intramedullary nails to fix tibial fractures.

In cases of open fracture or neurovascular compromise, urgent admission to theatre is needed for washout and exploration.

**Complications**  Common complications of tibial fractures are:

- compartment syndrome
- leg length discrepancy
- valgus or varus deformity
- non-union or malunion

Proximal tibial metaphyseal fractures can lead to late development of a valgus deformity at the knee.

# 11.13 Non-accidental injuries

A non-accidental injury is an injury purposefully inflicted by others, or knowingly not prevented by a person in charge of the injured child.

To distinguish an accidental from a non-accidental injury, it is essential to ensure a correlation between the mechanism of injury reported by the parent or carer and the pattern of the injury, and that there are no inconsistencies in the history. Missed non-accidental injury carries a 20% risk of further injury and a 5% chance of permanent neurological injury or death.

## Epidemiology

Non-accidental injuries are encountered in all socioeconomic groups. However, the incidence is higher in children with learning difficulties and children living in poverty.

Between 5 and 7% of children are neglected at home for various reasons, including parental drug and alcohol misuse, and this can lead to avoidable injuries. An estimated 8% of children are victims of abuse by a parent or carer.

Of all fractures caused by non-accidental injury, 80% are in children younger than 2 years.

## Clinical features

Many factors raise the suspicion of non-accidental injury. The following are red flags:

- inconsistencies in the history, or unexplained injuries
- delay in seeking medical attention for injuries
- a child's withdrawn demeanour or abnormal behaviour
- multiple injuries or fractures at differing stages of healing
- a fracture in a child who does not walk
- unusual injuries, for example cigarette burns, posterior rib fractures, bite marks or grip marks
- bruising in unusual places, such as the abdomen, buttocks, ears, fingertips or genitals

Other possible causes of the injury must be excluded, such as osteogenesis imperfecta (see page 341), leukaemia and renal disease. Mongolian blue spot is a birthmark that resembles bruising. A thorough examination and clear, concise documentation are required.

## Investigations

A full skeletal survey would show any old or healing fractures, and is warranted to detect any previous injuries. Fractures more likely to be caused by non-accidental injury are skull fractures, bilateral limb fractures, lateral clavicular fractures and sternal or scapular fractures.

## Management

An attempt is made to obtain the history from the child by interviewing them without the parent or carer being present. A parent's or carer's refusal to allow this is another red flag for non-accidental injury.

If there is any doubt about a diagnosis of non-accidental injury, the case must be discussed with a senior colleague. Child services are contacted, as well as the paediatric team. The priority is to prevent further harm to the child. The fracture is treated as appropriate.

# 11.14 Osteogenesis imperfecta

Osteogenesis imperfecta is a genetic disorder that results in either a decreased amount or an abnormal supply of type I collagen. This prevents the formation of good-quality bone and normal remodelling, and thereby leads to poor fracture healing, frequent fractures, insufficient remodelling and bone bowing. The condition is also associated with hearing, visual and dental problems.

## Epidemiology

The condition affects 6 or 7 people in 100,000.

## Causes

Osteogenesis imperfecta is usually caused by mutations in genes encoding type I collagen. It is inherited in an autosomal dominant or recessive manner.

There are eight types of osteogenesis imperfecta, which vary in severity. Type 2 is fatal shortly after birth, with death usually the result of respiratory problems and multiple fractures. Type 1 is the most common and mildest form of osteogenesis imperfecta; normal type I collagen is produced but in insufficient quantities.

### Clinical features

Children are typically shorter than their peers with limb deformities. Scoliosis, brittle teeth, a barrel ribcage and tinted, bluish sclera are common. Patients occasionally have respiratory problems.

### Investigations

Bone mineral density is measured. Genetic screening and collagen biopsy are also used to support a diagnosis.

### Management

There is no cure for osteogenesis imperfecta, so the aim of management is to prevent or reduce pain. The patient is encouraged to stay active to maintain muscle strength.

Fractures occur with mild or even no trauma. If there is clinical suspicion of a fracture, it is treated as such. This is done to limit the amount of radiation the child is exposed to, i.e. to minimise the number of X-rays taken. A healthy diet is encouraged, and blood tests are performed to ensure that the patient has normal levels of vitamin D and calcium.

Respiratory failure and accidental trauma are the main causes of death of patients with osteogenesis imperfecta.

# Orthopaedic trauma

Trauma is injury of the musculoskeletal system: bones, soft tissue, joints, ligaments, tendons, muscles and nerves. Trauma is a significant cause of mortality, particularly in younger age groups. In general, death as a consequence of trauma occurs with a trimodal distribution: immediate, early and late. Immediate death occurs as a consequence of a fatal injury. Early death occurs within hours to days, as a consequence of exsanguination or brain injury. Late death occurs within weeks of the injury as a consequence of sepsis or multi-organ failure. Early aggressive management of patients with trauma improves outcomes, particularly in the early phase.

## 12.1 Clinical scenario

### Polytrauma

#### Background and history

A motorcyclist has had a head-on collision with a car at a combined speed of 80 mph. He sustains multiple injuries and reports chest, pelvic and right lower limb pain.

#### Examination

The patient is assessed in accordance with the Advanced Trauma Life Support (ATLS) protocol. His airway is found to be clear, and his cervical spine is immobilised. He has reduced air entry on the right side of his chest. His oxygen saturation is 94% on 15 L/min of oxygen administered through a non-rebreathe mask, and his respiratory rate is 22 breaths/min. His systolic blood pressure is 78 mmHg. He is tachycardic, with a strong pulse, and has a Glasgow coma scale score of 15.

His abdomen is soft and non-tender, with obvious abrasions on the right side of his pelvis. His right lower limb has an obvious deformity with multiple abrasions. He is able to move all four limbs, although movement of the right limb is severely limited by pain. He has good peripheral pulses and normal sensation throughout all four limbs.

## Differential diagnosis

Any of the following may be present, given the mechanism of injury and examination findings:

- cervical spine injury
- right-sided chest wall injury with or without haemothorax or pneumothorax
- pelvic fracture
- right lower limb fracture
- internal bleeding from any of the injuries listed above

Common injuries from road traffic accidents include cervical spine injuries, haemothorax or pneumothorax and chest wall injuries, pelvic fractures and lower limb fractures. Many other fractures and soft tissue injuries are also possible.

> ### Clinical insight
>
> Consider the mechanism of injury and have a high index of suspicion for multiple injuries. With a mechanism of injury such as a high-speed collision, consider internal injuries from deceleration, hyperextension and hyperflexion.
>
> When treating a patient who has had a motorcycle accident, ascertain what protective clothing they were wearing and the state of that clothing after the accident; look at the helmet especially. Consider the structure of any vehicle involved in a road traffic accident. For example, on a motorbike the fuel tank sits directly in front of the pelvis, and in a car the airbag deploys directly in front of the chest wall and face.

## Investigations

The patient undergoes basic resuscitation in the emergency department. This includes administration of fluids or blood products, depending on the patient's grade of shock.

When stable, he will require a trauma CT scan of the head, cervical spine, chest, abdomen and pelvis. The CT findings, coupled with the clinical findings, will enable identification of any life-threatening injuries. Also when he is stable, anteroposterior and lateral radiographs of his lower limb injuries will be required. Each injury is initially managed and stabilised in the emergency department, with input and guidance from relevant specialties, when needed.

If necessary, the patient will undergo reduction of any bony injuries to ensure minimal neurovascular compromise. Fractures will to be stabilised with a simple back slab or splint. If there is any concern about the patient's neurovascular status, regular neurovascular re-examination of the right limb will be required.

## 12.2 Advanced Trauma Life Support

Advanced Trauma Life Support (ATLS) is a training programme designed to teach doctors how to systematically assess and treat patients with acute trauma. A primary survey is an overall assessment of the patient to look for any life-threatening injuries. This is done using a simple ABCDE approach.

### A. Airway and cervical spine:

- Is the patient talking?
- Are there any added sounds?
- Are there any foreign bodies in the airway?
- Is there any neck pain?

The cervical spine is immobilised with a hard collar, blocks and tape (triple immobilisation). If the mechanism of injury gives rise to concerns about the neck, triple immobilisation is put in place regardless of pain or clinical signs.

### B. Breathing:

- What is the patient's respiratory rate?
- What are their oxygen saturation values?
- Are there any abnormalities in the chest wall movements?
- Are their breath sounds normal?
- Are there any signs of a flail chest, or haemothorax or pneumothorax?

### C. Circulation:

- What is the patients' heart rate?
- What is their blood pressure?
- Do their peripheries feel cool or warm?
- Is there any obvious source of the patient's blood loss?

**D. Disability:**

- What is the patient's Glasgow coma scale score?
- What is their blood glucose concentration?

**E. Exposure:**

- Assess the abdomen
- Are there bowel sounds?
- Is there any pain?
- Is any blood present at the external urethral meatus?
- Is there any gross neurological deficit or deformity of any of the four limbs?

When exposing the patient's body for examination, always be aware of their temperature. It is best to keep them as covered and as warm as possible to avoid hypothermia.

Acute trauma patients typically have a serious injury causing severe pain. This may distract them, and the doctor, from other injuries. Therefore a systematic approach is used for the assessment, to ensure that nothing is missed.

Once the patient has been fully resuscitated and is stable, a secondary survey is done. This uses a more detailed approach, going from top to toe, looking for other injuries that may have occurred.

---

# 12.3 Open fractures

An open fracture is any fracture with a direct communication to a break in the skin. Open fractures are any fracture with a direct communication to a break in the skin. This includes perforation of a hollow viscus, for example penetration of the rectum by a pelvic fracture. An open fracture carries a higher risk of infection and complication. All open fractures require careful and timely management. Generally, open fractures are considered high energy injuries with a significant soft tissue component.

## Epidemiology

With open fractures, there is a wide distribution in both patients and fracture types and severity. Common fracture patterns encountered in open fractures are transverse tibial fractures, comminution, segmental fractures and bone loss. Multiple severe open fractures are most common in younger male patients, whereas isolated open fractures are more commonly caused by low-energy injuries in the elderly, particularly women. A third of patients with open fractures have polytrauma.

## Causes

Mechanisms of injury vary considerably, from simple falls in the elderly to high-energy trauma, for example from road traffic accidents, in the younger population.

## Clinical features

Patients present with pain, swelling, clinical deformity and loss of function. Patients have one or more wounds, which vary in size and appearance from small puncture wounds to larger wounds with visible bone and muscle injury and loss of soft tissue, which may be extensive (degloving).

The Gustilo–Anderson classification (**Table 12.1**) is commonly used to grade open fracture wounds. However, accurate grading is possible only after initial thorough debridement in the operating theatre. It should be appreciated that high-energy injuries carry a worse prognosis than low energy injuries even if the wound appears benign initially.

## Investigations

Radiographs and CT scans are obtained to assess the fracture pattern. Blood tests are used to check blood count and look

| Grade | Description |
|-------|-------------|
| I | Clean wound < 1 cm |
| II | Wound > 1 cm without extensive soft tissue damage |
| IIIA | Wound > 10 cm with soft tissue damage or crush injury; soft tissue coverage of bone should be possible |
| IIIB | Wound > 10 cm with extensive soft tissue damage and skin loss; usually requires soft tissue reconstruction |
| IIIC | Wound > 10 cm with extensive soft tissue damage and skin loss plus vascular injury; may require soft tissue reconstruction |

**Table 12.1** Gustilo–Anderson classification of open fracture wounds.

for inflammatory markers or signs of underlying illness. Vascular imaging is carried out if vascular injury is suspected.

## Management

The patient is initially assessed in accordance with the ATLS protocol, and resuscitated if necessary. Once they are haemo-dynamically stable, a systematic examination of the limb and open fracture is carried out as part of the secondary survey. Specifically, the fracture is reduced and stabilised or splinted, if necessary.

Neurovascular status is assessed and documented; this is repeated at varying intervals depending on severity of injury and clinical signs and symptoms. The wound is assessed and any gross contamination removed. It is photographed before being covered in a saline-soaked dressing.

Broad-spectrum intravenous antibiotics are administered, ideally within 3 h of injury, in accordance with local protocol. Tetanus vaccine is also administered. Once this is done, the patient undergoes further investigations, including imaging of the fracture. Urgent surgery is required to debride and wash out the wound, and the fracture is stabilised.

Reasons for immediate surgery include:
- gross contamination of the wound by marine, agricultural or sewage matter
- compartment syndrome
- vascular injury
- polytrauma

**Surgical management**  Non-operative management is not used, because all patients with open fracture require treatment in theatre for systematic and thorough debridement of the wound and stabilisation of the fracture. The fracture may be managed with definitive fixation primarily, or it may require temporary stabilisation, for example with external fixation, depending on the extent and size of the soft tissue injury.

A plastic surgery team is required for the management of open fractures and will be present in theatre ideally at the initial debridement. If the wound is not amenable to closing at first, another means of soft tissue coverage may be required, for example a skin flap or skin graft. Management of open fractures follows specific hospital and national guidelines.

The patient may have to return to theatre on multiple occasions, depending on the number and severity of their injuries.

### Complications
Open fractures are associated with the following complications:
- wound complications
- skin loss
- infection
- non-union
- neurovascular injury
- non-salvageable limb necessitating amputation

## 12.4 Compartment syndrome

Compartment syndrome is an orthopaedic emergency; although rare, it must not be missed. It is a limb- and life-threatening condition in which the circulation and function of tissues within a closed space are compromised by increased pressure within that space.

Muscles in a limb are contained within osseo-fascial compartments. These compartments are encapsulated by fascia which is inelastic. The condition develops because compartments have a relatively fixed volume. A small increase in pressure within a compartment shuts down the small low pressure venous system in the muscle, rapidly stopping outflow. Constriction by tight dressings or a cast further impairs outflow. Tissue perfusion is reduced which causes muscle and nerve ischaemia (**Figure 12.1**). If untreated, compartment syndrome leads to permanent damage to these structures.

### Epidemiology
The incidence of compartment syndrome is about 1 in 10,000 male patients and 7 in 10,000 female patients.

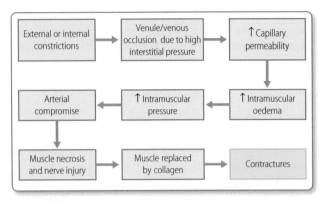

**Figure 12.1** The path linking muscle ischaemia to contractures.

## Causes

Compartment syndrome most commonly occurs after trauma. Tibial shaft and forearm fractures account for the greatest percentage of cases. Other causes include:

- orthopaedic surgery
- crush injuries
- vascular injury
- intensive muscle use or exercise
- snakebites
- gunshot wounds
- tourniquet use
- surgical positioning
- casting
- bleeding disorders
- infection
- non-union

About 10% of patients who develop compartment syndrome are on oral anticoagulants.

## Clinical features

The most consistent and reliable clinical symptom is pain that is disproportionate to that expected from the injury; the use of apparently adequate analgesia fails to manage the pain. Passive stretch of muscles contained within the compartment in question causes pain.

Other signs to look for are the five P's of acute ischaemia:

- pain
- paralysis
- pulselessness
- paraesthesia
- pallor

Pulselessness, paraesthesia and pallor are late signs; the limb is usually unsalvageable by the time they appear.

Diagnosis of compartment syndrome based on the 5 P's is unreliable. Compartment syndrome is always considered in cases of severe pain that is disproportionate to that expected for the injury sustained.

### Investigations

Compartment syndrome is a clinical diagnosis. However, pressure measurements are made if symptoms are subjective, or the patient is unconscious or has had regional anaesthesia. Various types of pressure monitor are used to measure compartment pressures; this should be done by an experienced senior colleague. Compartment pressures within 30 mmHg of diastolic blood pressure indicate compartment syndrome.

### Management

There is no conservative management for compartment syndrome. However, the following can be done on the ward:

- Ensure that the patient is normotensive, because hypotension worsens ischaemia
- Remove casts or constricting dressings
- Give supplemental oxygen to increase oxygen saturation
- Provide analgesia

**Surgical management** The patient requires emergency fasciotomy to release the pressure before permanent damage occurs. All the osseofascial compartments must be decompressed.

Indications for fasciotomy include:
- clinically suspected compartment syndrome
- pressure within 30 mmHg of diastolic blood pressure
- increasing tissue pressure
- significant tissue injury or a patient who already has a low threshold for intervention due to high risk of compartment syndrome
- >6 hours of total limb ischaemia
- injury associated with high risk of compartment syndrome
- neurovascular injury

The wounds are dressed but left open, and the patient is returned to theatre in 48–72 h. They are likely to require multiple further surgical procedures, usually with plastic surgery input to close or cover the wounds.

**Complications** Compartment syndrome has disastrous consequences if not recognised and treated appropriately and promptly. Complications can vary depending on the compartment effected. The most common complications are:
- cosmetic deformity
- permanent nerve damage
- infection
- loss of the limb
- death

## 12.5 Vascular injuries

Wounds and fractures involving vascular structures are surgical emergencies and require urgent exploration. The aim is to restore circulation within 3–4 h. Vascular surgeons are contacted immediately in cases of suspected vascular injury.

### Epidemiology

Vascular injuries are rare, but it is crucial that they are not missed. Any fracture or dislocation has the capacity to cause vascular injury. However, it is most commonly associated with open fractures and high-energy injuries, for example knee dislocations (up to 15% of which have associated vascular injury) and supracondylar fractures (1% of which have associated vascular injury).

## Causes

Causes of vascular injuries are:

- open fractures
- dislocations
- stab wounds
- gunshot wounds
- crush injuries

## Clinical features

The patient may have an open haemorrhaging wound

or obvious haematoma. If there is no wound, the fractured limb is usually cool and pale, with absent pulses and poor capillary refill. Frequent reassessment is required because any progression or change may alter the management and occasionally is an indication for emergency surgery. The rate and timing for reassessment will be dictated by the patient's individual circumstances. Ankle–brachial pressure index (ABPI) values are obtained if signs of vascular compromise are present.

## Investigations

If a pulse is not palpable, Doppler ultrasound is used to confirm whether or not it is absent. An angiogram (**Figure 12.2**) is obtained if vascular injury, with or without embolisation, is suspected.

## Management

Initial treatment is in accordance with the ATLS protocol. Direct pressure is applied over any obvious haemorrhaging wound. Circulation must be restored for the limb to survive. The fracture or dislocation is reduced and immobilised, and vascular status reassessed. If a vessel has been kinked as a result of displacement of the fracture or dislocation, reduction usually restores circulation in closed injuries. If reduction fails to produce any improvement, exploration of the vessels is required.

**Surgical management**  In vascular injury, the patient is likely to require urgent operative management, and vascular surgeons must be contacted as soon as possible. In theatre, internal or

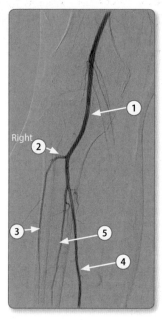

**Figure 12.2** Digital subtraction angiogram of the popliteal artery ① as it trifurcates ② into vessels supplying the leg and foot: the anterior tibial artery ③, the posterior tibial artery ④ and the peroneal artery ⑤.

external fixation of a fracture is usually carried out first, followed by the vascular procedure.

**Complications** The complications of vascular injuries are:
- neurological symptoms
- muscle necrosis
- loss of limb
- death

# Orthopaedic infections and other soft tissue problems

chapter
13

Orthopaedic structures can either be the primary source of infection or become involved secondary to an infection, usually via haematogenous spread.

Most infections are treated with antibiotics, however the presence of pus or an abscess requires surgical drainage, and dead bone or an infected implant will require surgery. Removing the source of infection (source control), often with surgery and systemic antibiotics, is also a strategy used to manage infections.

The most commonly seen organisms in orthopaedic infections are the patient's own skin commensals, usually *Staphylococcus* or *Streptococcus*. *Pseudomonas aeruginosa* is often present in more prolonged infections. In patients with diabetes, vascular disease or who are immunocompromised, Gram-negative and anaerobic bacteria are most commonly seen, particularly in the lower leg or foot.

Always seek the advice of an infectious disease specialist when managing orthopaedic infections.

## 13.1 Clinical scenario

### Acutely painful shoulder

#### Background

A 44-year-old woman is seen in the emergency department with an acutely painful right shoulder. She did a strenuous session in the gym 2 days ago. She had put the pain down to a muscular strain but is now feeling hot, feverish and nauseated.

#### History

The patient is otherwise well, with no notable past medical history and no history of trauma. She has had no operations on her right shoulder. It occasionally becomes stiff and achy, but this resolves spontaneously after a day or two.

### Examination

The patient looks flushed and is pyrexial, with a temperature of 38.5°. She has a marked decrease in the range of movement of her right shoulder, which also appears erythematous. All other joints are normal. Joint aspiration results in a 'dry tap' (an aspiration that does not yield a sample).

Radiographs appear normal. However, blood tests show a C-reactive protein concentration of 213 mg/L (normal <5 mg/L) and a white cell count of 16 x$10^9$/L (normal 4.00–11.0 x$10^9$/L).

### Differential diagnosis

Possible causes of the patient's shoulder pain are:
- septic arthritis
- cellulitis
- necrotising fasciitis
- supraspinatus tendonitis
- musculoskeletal tenderness and concurrent infection
- acute calcific tendinitis

Given this patient is pyrexial with raised inflammatory markers and a reduced range of movement, septic arthritis is the most likely diagnosis. The patient undergoes an arthroscopic washout of the shoulder and pus is found in the joint. Her condition improves and she has a subsequent washout 48 hours later. She makes a full recovery following a 6-week course of flucloxacillin.

## 13.2 Septic arthritis

Septic arthritis is an infection in a joint space, usually in the knee. If untreated, or if treatment is delayed, septic arthritis leads to extensive, permanent cartilage damage. The damage may start as early as 8 h into the infection, so septic arthritis is an orthopaedic surgical emergency.

### Epidemiology

Both native and prosthetic joints are affected. Septic arthritis affects 8 in 100,000 people and is more common in men. It has a higher incidence in the elderly and immunocompromised, and affects both native and prosthetic joints.

## Causes

The commonest causative organisms are skin commensals, usually *Staphylococcus aureus*. Other common organisms are *Neisseria gonorrhoea* in sexually active young adults, and *Escherichia coli* in the elderly and intravenous drug users.

## Clinical features

Patients with septic arthritis are typically systemically unwell, with a very painful, warm, erythematous joint; extremely reduced range of movement; and inability to weight-bear. Kocher's criteria are used to help identify cases of septic arthritis:

- non-weight-bearing
- erythrocyte sedimentation rate > 40 mm/h
- white cell count > 12 x $10^9$/L
- fever (temperature > 38.5°)

A point is given for each criterion met. The total score indicates the likelihood of the patient having septic arthritis (**Table 13.1**).

## Investigations

Required blood tests are blood cultures, erythrocyte sedimentation rate, C-reactive protein and full blood count. Anteroposterior and lateral radiographs and ultrasound scans of the affected joint may show joint space widening and an effusion, or they may appear normal (particularly in early infection).

| Score | Likelihood of septic arthritis (%) |
|:---:|:---:|
| 1 | 3 |
| 2 | 40 |
| 3 | 93 |
| 4 | 99 |

Table 13.1 Kocher's criteria: interpretation of score.

Fluid around the joint is aspirated, and the sample sent for Gram staining, cell count, cultures, crystals and glucose measurement. If the affected joint is prosthetic, aspiration must be carried out in a laminar flow operating theatre.

## Management

Intravenous antibiotics are started immediately after aspiration has been carried out, in line with local guidelines. The antibiotics used are changed, if necessary, when the results of sensitivity testing become available. Washout of the joint is carried out in theatre as soon as this is possible.

# 13.3 Osteomyelitis

Osteomyelitis is an infection of the bone with progressive inflammatory destruction. It occurs in three ways:
- haematogenous spread (the commonest mechanism)
- penetrating injury
- contiguous spread via soft tissue or ulceration

The condition is classified as acute (< 2 weeks), subacute (1–6 months) or chronic (> 6 months). It occasionally leads to infarction of the local bone and abscess formation. Infarcted bone, known as sequestrum, can form an encapsulated area impenetrable to the body's natural defences and antibiotics.

## Epidemiology

Osteomyelitis occurs more commonly in those living in developing countries, intravenous drug users, the elderly and diabetics. Trauma accounts for nearly half of reported cases of osteomyelitis worldwide.

## Causes

The infection is commonly caused by *S. aureus*. In patients with sickle cell disease, the causative organism is usually *Salmonella*.

Risk factors for osteomyelitis include diabetes, trauma, immunosuppression, poor blood supply and intravenous drug use.

## Clinical features

Osteomyelitis presents with pain, fever, erythema, discharge and a reduced range of movement in the adjacent joints. There is occasionally also a draining sinus.

In children, the usual presentation is with bone pain and fever. However, an acute presentation of leukaemia or bone tumour must be excluded because these conditions are life threatening and may present in a very similar manner to osteomyelitis.

## Investigations

Blood tests, i.e. C-reactive protein, erythrocyte sedimentation rate, full blood count, urea and electrolytes and blood cultures, are required to help confirm the diagnosis of infection or inflammation. A wound swab is also needed if there is a wound or discharge from which a sample can be obtained.

Radiographs may show a lytic or sclerotic lesion (**Figure 13.1**). MRI is especially effective for visualising soft tissue involvement. In cases of doubt, a tissue sample is obtained for biopsy; this will also be helpful for sensitivity testing.

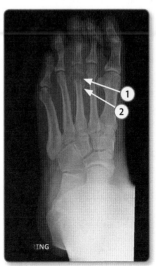

**Figure 13.1** Anteroposterior radiograph showing osteomyelitis: infection of the 3rd metatarsal in a patient with diabetic foot. Lysis ① is a consequence of bony destruction. New subperiosteal bone has formed involucrum ②.

## Management

Osteomyelitis is primarily treated non-operatively with long-term antibiotics. However, if the patient does not have an adequate response to antibiotics, bony and soft tissue debridement is necessary. Subsequent debridement may be necessary after the index surgery, to ensure removal of all infected tissue.

**Conservative management** This requires long-term use of antibiotics. It may be possible to treat osteomyelitis completely with the use of appropriate antibiotics for ≥ 3 months.

Patients with chronic osteomyelitis or who are unsuitable candidates for surgery usually need to take antibiotics indefinitely to suppress the underlying infection. However, long-term antibiotic use may fail to treat the condition completely in these patients and they risk flare ups of the disease returning, which may become life threatening if systemic sepsis occurs.

**Surgical management** Operative treatment consists of thorough debridement of infected material, both bony and soft tissue. Antibiotics are used for up to 6 months after surgery.

The principle of treatment is to cure the infection and allow the bone to heal.

## 13.4 Gangrene

Gangrene is tissue death resulting from severe vascular compromise. It is a sign of critical ischaemia.

The condition typically presents in the peripheries, i.e. the fingers and toes. However, it can develop in any part of the body, including the internal organs.

### Epidemiology

Gangrene is more common in diabetics and smokers due to the poor vascular supply.

## Causes

Gangrene is typically caused by trauma, peripheral vascular disease or any chronic condition resulting in vascular compromise. Risk factors include smoking and diabetes.

## Clinical features

Gangrene is described as 'wet' or 'dry'.
- In wet gangrene, a bacterial infection is present in the affected tissue
- In dry gangrene, the affected tissue is not infected

The prognosis is better with dry rather than wet gangrene.

In wet gangrene, the skin appears bruised, erythematous and painful, and blisters and pus may be present. If septic, the patient may be pyrexial, tachycardic and hypotensive, and they may have altered mental status and reduced urine output.

## Investigations

Wound swab samples are obtained. If the patient is systemically unwell, an arterial blood gas to check for lactate and acidosis as well as blood cultures are required. Other blood tests, including full blood count, C-reactive protein measurement and urea and electrolytes, are useful to determine the severity of the infection, assess the response to treatment and monitor for renal failure.

## Management

Treatment depends on the location of the gangrene and its severity. Early involvement of the vascular team is essential so that revascularisation can be attempted.

In cases of sepsis, particularly in the presence of wet gangrene, surgical debridement, with or without amputation, is carried out

> ### Clinical insight
>
> Gas gangrene, also known as clostridial myonecrosis, is a form of gangrene caused by infection with the Gram-positive anaerobe *Clostridium perfringens*. Release of a gas biproduct of the infection results in surgical emphysema in the surrounding tissues.
>
> Treatment is urgent radical debridement. Gas gangrene with bacteraemia has 50% mortality. Death is usually the result of overwhelming sepsis causing shock and renal failure.

without delay. Antibiotics are always administered, in line with local guidelines. If the gangrene is mild or the patient is not well enough for surgery, then appropriate wound care, the use of dressings, and elevation of the affected tissue are all advised.

## 13.5 Necrotising fasciitis

Necrotising fasciitis is a rapidly progressive, life-threatening infection that spreads through the soft tissue planes. It spares the deep fascia and muscle.

### Epidemiology

Necrotising fasciitis typically occurs in patients in their late 30s, and is more common in men. It can occur after surgical or medical procedures, trauma, insect bites and intramuscular injections. Risk factors include obesity, immunosuppression, diabetes, intravenous drug use, high alcohol intake and cancer.

### Causes

Between 85 and 90% of cases of necrotising fasciitis are poly-microbial; causative organisms include both anaerobic and aerobic organisms.

### Clinical features

Patients with necrotising fasciitis appear very unwell, with signs of severe sepsis. They typically have pain, pyrexia and rigors, and rapidly progressing skin changes. The condition is associated with cellulitis. The skin appears discoloured and has a woody, tense feel to it.

### Investigations

Blood samples are obtained immediately before antibiotics are started, and sent for tests including cultures. Administration of antibiotics must not be delayed until the results become available.

A sample of affected tissue can be biopsied to identify the causative organism (or organisms), but again, treatment should not be delayed by the wait for results.

| Result | Score |
|---|---|
| C-reactive protein > 150 mg/L | 4 |
| White cell count (x 10⁹/L) | |
| 15–25 | 1 |
| > 25 | 2 |
| Haemoglobin (g/dL) | |
| 11–13.5 | 1 |
| < 11 | 2 |
| Sodium < 135 mmol/L | 2 |
| Creatinine > 141 μmol/L | 2 |
| Glucose > 10 mmol/L | 1 |
| A total score > 6 has a positive predictive value for necrotising fasciitis of 92%. | |

**Table 13.2** Laboratory Risk Indicator for Necrotising Fasciitis scoring system.

Mortality is significantly reduced the shorter the time until surgery. Mortality ranges from 20–80%.

The Laboratory Risk Indicator for Necrotising Fasciitis scoring system is used to calculate the likelihood of necrotising fasciitis in individual cases (**Table 13.2**).

### Management

The patient is admitted to emergency theatre for radical surgical debridement; amputation is considered in cases of irreversible necrosis and severe sepsis. Long-term use of broad-spectrum antibiotics is required.

## 13.6 Postoperative wound infections

Closure of operative wounds occurs in one of two ways:
- by primary intention, when the edges are opposed and the wound is closed with sutures, staples, adhesive tape or glue
- secondary intention, when the wound is left open and allowed to heal by itself

Postoperative wound infection occurs at the surgical site and has a detrimental effect on wound healing. It also offers a route of infection deeper into neighbouring tissues, including bones and joints.

### Epidemiology and causes

Postoperative wound infection usually occurs within 30 days of the skin surface being breeched. Risk factors include patients who are immunocompromised, diabetics, smokers, patients who are taking steroids or are obese. After traumatic injury, 15% of operative wounds become infected.

### Clinical features

Typical features include pain, erythema and discharge at the site of a postoperative wound, as well as fever and malaise.

### Investigations

Radiographs of the affected area are needed, to look especially for non-union if there had been a fracture. MRI scans are helpful to visualise the soft tissues in cases of doubt. Blood tests, including cultures, are required to assess inflammation and infection. A wound swab sample is sent for microbiological tests.

### Management

It is usually possible to treat postoperative wound infections conservatively with antibiotics.

If the conservative approach is not possible, management is with washout and debridement, as well as long-term antibiotic use. Metalwork, if present, is occasionally removed if the fracture site is stable, but it is best left in place if the fracture site is unstable.

## 13.7 Cellulitis

Cellulitis is an inflammatory, non-necrotising superficial skin infection. There is no deep component to the infection, i.e. there are no abscesses or ulceration, although these can be present concurrently.

### Epidemiology

Cellulitis occurs equally in men and women and is more common in people over 45 years of age. It is more common in the elderly, diabetics, and those who are immunocompromised.

### Causes

Cellulitis is usually the result of a staphylococcal infection. It can occur anywhere in the body but usually develops on the legs. Oedematous tissue, areas of trauma and operation sites are at particular risk.

### Clinical features

The superficial skin appears erythematous and warm, with swelling and tenderness. Patients can be systemically well or unwell, and treatment is targeted accordingly. If patients are systematically unwell they may need to be admitted for IV antibiotics, whereas if patients are otherwise well they can be treated as an outpatient with oral antibiotics.

### Investigations

Blood tests are required to detect signs of systemic illness and to monitor the course of the infection. Blood and wound swab samples may also be needed for cultures.

If the cellulitis is mild, few or no investigations are necessary. However, blood tests are useful for monitoring.

### Management

Antibiotic treatment is required, along with wound care. Control of diabetes is essential if this is the underlying disorder.

## 13.8 Abscesses

An abscess is a localised collection of pus. Any area of the body can be affected, but the axilla, natal cleft and groin are the most common sites. Abscesses frequently occur on the feet of patients with diabetes. The most common cause is infection by methicillin-resistant *S. aureus* (MRSA).

### Epidemiology

Abscesses are very common and occur in any age group. They can appear on any part of the body and usually require incision and drainage.

### Causes

Abscesses can be due to either blocked glands, insect bites or other small breaks in the skin which create a route for infection. Risk factors include diabetic patients, patients who are immunocompromised, intravenous drug users and alcoholics.

### Clinical features

The abscess starts as a small, hard, painful collection of pus. This then enlarges, softens and becomes fluctuant. If left untreated, it discharges its contents via the route of least resistance; this can result in a fistula.

Patients occasionally complain of local pain and swelling. If they have become systemically unwell, they additionally present with a swinging fever, tachycardia and lethargy.

### Investigations

If the patient is systemically unwell, blood tests are done to assess the severity of the infection and to monitor its course. Blood and swab samples are sent for cultures to ensure that the appropriate antibiotics are used. US is useful if the abscess is suspected to be communicating with surrounding spaces or structures, or to confirm the diagnosis if there is doubt.

### Management

Surgical drainage is required, because antibiotics are unable to sufficiently penetrate the fibrous capsule surrounding the abscess. However, antibiotics are given if the patient is unable or unwilling to undergo surgery, this can lead to a prolonged healing time and occasionally a chronic ulcer. It can also occasionally lead to worsening and further progression of the disease.

## 13.9 Foot ulcers

An ulcer is an abnormal break in the epithelial layer. The most common cause of foot ulcers in the UK is neuropathy as a consequence of diabetes.

All ulcers are initially colonised by skin commensal bacteria. If left untreated the ulcer deepens, allowing bacteria to enter deeper tissues causing osteomyelitis, abscess formation and chronic infection. This is consequently both limb- and life-threatening. Other causes of foot ulcers include chronic neurological conditions, vascular disease (both venous and arterial) and decubitus ulceration (pressure ulceration usually affecting the heel).

Given the potential for significant harm, all foot ulceration should be taken seriously.

### Causes

Most foot ulcers occur in patients with diabetes, in whom they are a chronic problem leading to higher rates of morbidity and mortality. The loss of sensation associated with diabetes means that insults to the foot go unnoticed and the resulting wounds worsen with repetitive trauma. Poor wound healing also contributes to the development of foot ulcers in diabetic patients.

Risk factors include high alcohol intake, smoking, poor nutrition and poor circulation. Ulcers are associated with osteomyelitis, cellulitis and infection. Any cause of neuropathy predisposes an individual to ulceration to the foot.

An estimated 85% of lower limb amputations are carried out because of ulcers. However, ulcers are usually managed medically.

### Clinical features

The ulcer is often a painless, well-demarcated lesion with possible discharge and local erythema. The skin typically appears necrotic or infected (**Figure 13.2**).

To ensure that no ulcers are missed, examination must include both feet, with inspection of the areas between the toes.

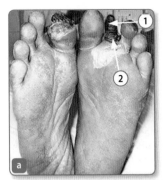

**Figure 13.2** (a) Note black discoloration ① and clear-cut line of demarcation ②.
(b) Diabetic foot with significant neuroischaemic ulceration. The ulceration is deep, almost certainly down to the bone.

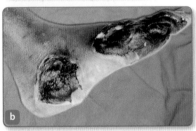

Ulcer formation is often multi-factorial; usually multiple mechanisms of ulceration are present to greater or lesser degrees.

*Diabetic patients* Pressure is usually the initiating factor in diabetic patients, however, small vessel disease with relative hypoxia prevents the skin from healing. A change in foot shape as a consequence of motor neuropathy, and scaly and dry skin as a consequence of autonomic neuropathy all cause ulcer formation.

*Vascular patients* Vascular patients develop ulceration due to areas of skin becoming critically ischaemic, either by arterial inflow being compromised or as a result of increased pressure due to venous insufficiency. Typically, arterial ulcers affect the digits and venous ulceration affects the ankle.

*Bed-bound patients*  Bed-bound patients are prone to ulcers at areas of pressure to the feet, usually where their heels rest on the mattress.

### Investigations

Anteroposterior and lateral radiographs are obtained to look for evidence of osteomyelitis. If further imaging is required, MRI is the gold standard for visualising soft tissues. Bloods tests are done to look for increased levels of inflammatory markers and to monitor infection. If the patient is systemically unwell or has sepsis, wound swab and blood samples are obtained for cultures before antibiotics are given Ideally, a deep tissue biopsy should be taken at the time of any surgical intervention or when the diagnosis is unclear. Antibiotics should be withheld, where possible, until this sample is obtained.

### Management

Ulcers are usually managed medically by strict diabetic control, wound care, pressure relief (offloading), footwear alterations, patient education and long-term foot care. If infection is present, antibiotics are needed, as well as surgical debridement and in extreme cases amputation.

## 13.10 Foreign bodies

A foreign body lodging in tissue is usually a consequence of skin puncture; this is common in the hands and feet. A foreign body in the foot usually occurs as a consequence of treading on a sharp object. The patient may or may not recall such an incident. A foreign body in the hand often also occurs as a result of injury by a sharp object, e.g. a wood splinter or glass. Most patients present immediately with the retained foreign body. Some patients present later with chronic pain after an initial puncture some time previously. Pain is the common presenting feature of a chronic retained foreign body. There may or may not be evidence of infection.

In blast or high pressure injuries foreign material is literally forced through the skin.

### Epidemiology

In general, most foreign bodies are sharp and enter directly through the skin, e.g. wood, glass and metal splinters. Chronically, an abscess may form if the tissue around the foreign body becomes infected. Both granuloma and abscess will present with pain and swelling.

### Causes

Foreign bodies enter the body via various mechanisms. The most obvious of these is entry through breaches of the skin in cases of large open fractures. Foreign bodies can also enter the body via penetrating injuries (**Figure 13.3**), trauma caused by an explosion and direct self-harm.

### Clinical features

The patient may or may not be aware of a foreign body. If it is unnoticed, it may remain dormant or become infected over time and present with erythema and pain as an infected mass or collection of pus.

### Investigations

If a suspicion of a foreign body due to the mechanism of injury or puncture wounds a radiograph should be performed. Foreign bodies have varying degrees of radio-opacity. Metal and glass are seen well on radiographs. Wood is less reliably

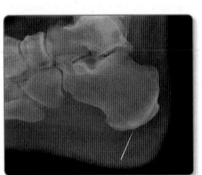

**Figure 13.3** Lateral radiograph of the heel, showing the presence of a needle. The patient had stepped on the needle while walking around his house barefoot.

detected on imaging. If the patient is a delayed presentation with signs of infection then inflammatory markers should be monitored.

## Management

Washout and excision of the foreign body is carried out, usually alongside the use of antibiotics. If the foreign body is particularly small or has been present for a long time without causing concern, it is possible for it to be left in place, with the patient advised to seek medical assistance if they notice any signs of infection. As a general principle, emergency management should ensure that the patient is adequately covered for tetanus and given boosters as appropriate, along with planning for removal of the foreign body.

# 13.11 Bite injuries

Human bite injuries are the third most common bite injuries behind cats and dogs. They have a high risk of infection and often present late as they are under-estimated by the patient. Transmission of infectious diseases can also occur with human bites so it is important to fully investigate and protect the patient as much as possible, including the use of anti-retrovirals if appropriate. Treatment involves reducing soft tissue damage and minimising infection.

## Epidemiology

Human bite injuries are most commonly of the hand, and about 15% become infected. They are a route of transmission for viruses such as hepatitis B and C, herpes simplex virus and tetanus.

Bite injuries usually present in young men as a result of an act of aggression. Up to 44% occur in men aged 16–25 years old.

## Causes

Bite injuries are often sustained during rough sexual encounters, domestic violence and close-contact sporting accidents. They are also encountered in cases of direct self-harm and child abuse. Bite injuries to the hand may be caused by the impact of a punch against another person's mouth.

### Clinical features

An accurate history is needed to enable appropriate treatment. Disclosure of the mechanism of injury is likely to take time to solicit if the patient's circumstances are especially sensitive, for example in cases of domestic violence or child abuse.

A puncture wound is present, which correlates with the history. In cases of late presentation, there may be obvious infection, with erythema and discharge.

If the patient has comorbidities resulting in immunocompromise, the wound must be monitored closely for signs of infection. If the wound was sustained in an assault, the patient's notes may be required as a legal report; photographic evidence is recommended.

### Investigations

The patient must always be asked about their vaccination status. This is important to ensure they have protection against possible transmission of infectious diseases.

Blood tests are carried out if there is clinical suspicion of infection or transmission of disease; a wound swab sample is also sent for microbiological tests. A radiograph is obtained if a fracture or foreign body is suspected.

### Management

The most common complications of bite injuries are functional deficit and scarring, as well as possible transmission of an infectious disease.

## 13.12 Neuropathic arthopathy

A neuropathic joint, otherwise known as Charcot's joint, is a weight-bearing joint with progressive degeneration. It can result in bony destruction, dislocation, fractures and deformity all of which can lead to significant disability. The exact pathophysiology is unknown and is likely to be to be multi-factorial. It is likely that repeated micro trauma to a neuropathic joint causes an amplification of bone and joint destruction by a positive feedback mechanism, resulting in an unchecked inflammatory response leading to significant neuro-arthropathy.

## Epidemiology

In high-income countries, the commonest cause is diabetes with peripheral neuropathy, and the joint most likely to be affected is the ankle. Charcot joint is usually unilateral, but up to 25% of cases are bilateral. Any condition causing neuropathy puts the patient at risk of neuropathic arthropathy. Alchohol is another common cause.

## Causes

Neuropathic arthropathy is the consequence of reduced sensation and abnormal proprioception, constituting a loss of the body's natural protective mechanism. This allows the condition to spiral into a loop of positive feedback where, instead of resting, the damaged joint is subjected to further and repeated injurious episodes. The exact mechanism remains unknown.

## Clinical features

Onset is slow and insidious. The affected joint is usually swollen but painless, with a reduced range of movement. It can be

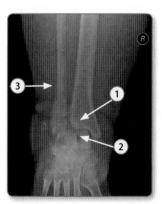

**Figure 13.4** Anteriorposterior radiograph showing neuropathic joint, in this case the right ankle, secondary to diabetic neuropathy. There is destruction of the normal architecture of the ankle ①, including destruction of the talus ②. A reactive periosteal response is visible at the distal fibula ③.

erythematous and warm to touch, which explains the frequent concern regarding possible infection. Instability and fragmentation lead to subluxation and deformity.

## Investigations

Radiographs of the affected joint are imperative; both antero-posterior and lateral views are required. Radiography usually shows florid destruction and fragmentation of the joint (**Figure 13.4**). The findings are usually so florid that a diagnosis of joint infection is erroneously diagnosed and treated with antibiotics; little else causes such a rapid and severe destructive picture.

Occasionally it may be difficult in diabetic patients to differentiate neuropathic joint from a joint infection. MRI may help in this instance, particularly if an abscess or a collection of fluid, blood or pus is visible on the scan. Blood tests show increased erythrocyte sedimentation rate and white cell count in cases of infection.

## Management

The key to successful management of a neuropathic joint is patient awareness and education, enabling patients to monitor and manage their condition.

A total contact cast is used to offload the joint and preserve the shape of the limb. The cast usually rapidly stabilises the condition and allows for resolution and healing. Strict monitoring of the cast is needed as the swelling reduces and the cast becomes looser.

Patients must be followed up to allow their condition to be monitored and their changing needs addressed. Long-term management with braces, orthotics and potentially surgery and amputation are all considered. Diabetic control needs to be optimised to prevent further deterioration.

# Index

Note: Page numbers in **bold** or *italic* refer to tables or figures respectively.

## A

ABCDE approach, for trauma patients 345–346
Abscesses 365–366
Acetabular fracture 232–236
    anteroposterior radiograph 233, *234*
    CT scan 233
    hip dislocation and 233
    iliac view 233, *234*
    Judet–Letournel classification 233, 235
    left *235*
    obturator view 233, *234*
Acetabulum 222
Achilles tendon ruptures 271–272, 297–299
Acromioclavicular joint 90, *91*
    injuries 102–103, *103*
Acromioclavicular ligament 90, *91*
Acromion *88*, 90
Advance directive 9
Advanced Trauma Life Support (ATLS) 345–346
Advance statement 8, 9
Amputation 54
Anatomical snuffbox 162, *163*
Angulation 3
Ankle arthrodesis 288
Ankle–brachial pressure index (ABPI) 353
Ankle fracture 279–285
    bimalleolar fractures 281
    Danis–Weber classification 281, **282**, *283*, *284*
    Lauge–Hansen classification 281–282
    mortise view radiograph 281, *281*
    open reduction and internal fixation 284, *285*
    Ottawa ankle rules 280, *280*
    stable fracture 282
    trimalleolar fractures 281
Ankle sprains 289–291
    grading of ligamentous injuries 289, **289**
    MRI in 290, *290*
    radiographs in 290
    RICE principles 290
Antalgic gait **29**
Anterior cruciate ligament, injury to 263–265, *264*
Anterior drawer test **33**, **34**, *248*
Anterior talofibular ligament 272
Anterior tibial artery 273
Antibiotics, use of 46
Apprehension test 107
Arthrocentesis *see* Joint aspiration
Arthrodesis 51–52
Arthroplasty 52–53
    excision 52
    hemireplacement 52
    total replacement 52–53
Articular fractures 2–3
Ataxic gait **29**
Avascular necrosis 293–294
Avulsion fractures 226 *see also* Pelvic fracture
Axillary artery 92, *92*
Axillary nerve 86, *86*, 92
Axonotmesis **14**

## B

Back pain 55–56
Barton fracture **156**
Base-of-thumb fractures 176–178, *177*
    Bennett fracture 176, *177*, *179*
    extra-articular fractures 176, *1/8*
    intra-articular fracture 176
    Rolando fracture 176, *177*

Beighton score for joint hypermobility 252, **253**
Bennett fractures 176, *177, 179*
Biceps tendon injuries 123–124
Bisphosphonates 46
Bite injuries 371–372
Blood tests **43**, 43–44
    blood transfusion 43–44
    infection markers 44
    microbiology 44
    specific markers 44
Bone grafting 53
Bone healing 4–5
Bony Bankart lesion 108
Bouchard's nodes **22**
Boutonnière deformity **23**
Boxer's fracture 170
Brachial artery 128, 319
Brachial plexus 92–93, *93*
    injuries 121–123
Bruising 25
Bulbocavernosus reflex 66
Burst fractures, of lumbar spine 72, *72, 73*

**C**
Cadaveric bone 53
Calcaneal fractures 294–297
    Böhler's angle 295, *296*
    classification 295
    CT scans 295, *296*
    lateral radiograph 295, *296*
    Mondor's sign 295
Calcaneal gait **29**
Calcaneofibular ligament 272
Calf squeeze test **34**, 271
Capacity 7
    assessment 8
    in children 9
    factors affecting 7–8
    lack of 8–9
Capitellum fractures 139–141, *141*
    anteroposterior radiograph 140, *141*
    classification 140
Caput ulna **23**
Carpal bones 148, *148*

Carpal keystone 166 *see also* Lunate dislocations
Carpometacarpal joints 148
Cauda equina 60
Cauda equina syndrome 56, 67–70
    atraumatic 67
    blood tests 70
    disc herniation and 67, 68
    MRI scan 69, *69*
    surgical decompression 70
    traumatic 67
Cellulitis 364–365
Cervical spine injuries 73
    C1 fractures 75, *75*
    C2 fractures 75–76, *76, 77*
    compression injuries 74
    extension injuries 74
    flexion injuries 73–74
    flexion-with-rotation injuries 74
    management 77
Chance fracture 72–73
Chauffeur's fracture **156**
Clavicle 87
Clavicular fractures 97, 99–102
    anteroposterior radiograph 100, *100*
    computerised tomography 100
    group I 97
    group II 97
    group III 97
    surgical management 100–101, *101*
    tenting of skin 99, *99*
Claw hand **22**
Claw toes **23**
Clostridial myonecrosis *see* Gas gangrene
Coccygeal fractures 238
Collateral ligament stability testing 246, *247*
Colles fracture **156**, 160
Compartment syndrome 171, 349–352, *350*
Complex regional pain syndrome type 1 160
Computerised tomography 38–39
    advantages/disadvantages 39, **39**

principles 38–39
terminology 39
Condylar fractures 322–327
CRITOL (mnemonic) 325, **325**
lateral condylar fractures 323, *323*
medial epicondylar fracture 323, *324, 326*
paediatric elbow, anatomy of *326*
Consent 6
capacity to 7–9
expressed verbal 6
expressed written 6
implied 6
informed 7
voluntary 7
Conservative management 45–46
Coracoclavicular ligament 90, *91*
Coracoid processes *88*, 90
Coronoid process fractures 144–145
Cruciate ligament testing 246, *248*
Cytotoxic drugs 46

**D**
Deep peroneal nerve 273, *276*, **277**, *277*
Deformities 22, **22–23**
Deltoid ligament 272
Diagnostic categories 21, **21**
Dislocation 3–4
elbow 131–134, *132*
hip 193–197
knee 267–269
patella 252–253
shoulder 85–87, 106–111
Displacements 3
angulation 3
distraction and impaction 3
rotation 3
translation and shortening 3
Distal femoral fractures 259–261, *260*
Distal humerus fractures *see* Supracondylar fractures
Distal radioulnar joint (DRUJ) 160
injuries 160–162, *161*
ligaments of *161*
Distal radius fractures **156**, 156–160, *157, 158, 159*

classification of **156**
fixation 159, *159*
lateral radiograph *158*
malreduced 160
posteroanterior radiograph *157*
Drug history 19

**E**
Elbow 125, *127*
articulations and ligaments *127*, 127–128
capitellum fractures 139–141, *141*
coronoid process fractures 144–145
dislocations 131–134, *132*
examination 128–130, *130*
innervation 128, *129*
lateral epicondylitis 126, 145–146
medial epicondylitis 146
movements 130, *130*
olecranon *127*, 128
olecranon bursitis 145
olecranon fractures 137–139, *138, 139*
pain 125–126
radial head and neck fractures 141–144, *143*
supracondylar fractures 134–136, *135, 136*
vascular supply 128
Epiphyseal fractures, in children 338
Erb–Duchenne palsy 122
Essex-Lopresti fracture 161
Examination
anatomical measurements 32, 34–35, *35*
beginning of 28
fracture and dislocation assessment 35
gait 28, **29**
general examination 28
joint examination 28–32, **33–34**
neurovascular status of limb 36
trauma assessment and management 35–36
traumatic vs non-traumatic 28

**F**

Falls  19
Family history  20
Fasciotomy  352
Femoral head fractures  218
Femoral shaft fractures
    anteroposterior radiograph  *210*
    in children  335–338, **337**, *337*
    intramedullary nailing  211, *212*
Fixed flexion  26
Fixed flexion deformities (FFD)  **23**,
    26–27
Flexor tendon sheath infection  182–183
Foot and ankle  271
    Achilles tendon ruptures  271–272,
        297–299
    ankle fracture  279–285
    ankle joint movement  *278*
    ankle sprains  289–291
    bones and ligaments  272, *273*,
        *274, 275*
    calcaneal fractures  294–297
    examination  274–276
    foot and toes movement  *278*
    innervation  273, *276*, **277**, *277*
    Lisfranc injuries  300–302
    metatarsal fractures  303–308
    navicular fractures  310–311
    phalangeal fractures  308–310
    pilon fracture  285–288
    plantar fasciitis  311
    surface anatomy  *273, 274, 274, 275*
    talus fractures  291–294
    vascular supply  273, *276, 277*
Foot drop  196
Foot ulcers  367–369, *368*
Foreign body, in foot  311
Fracture  1
    articular vs nonarticular  2–3
    closed vs open  1–2
    dislocations  3–4
    displacement  3
    healing and complications  4–6
    patterns  1, *2*
    simple vs comminuted  2

Fracture management  46–51
    devices for, use of  49–51
    local anaesthetic  51
    questions in  **47–48**
    reduction and stabilisation  48–49
    stable fracture  48

**G**

Gait  21, 271
    examination of  28
    types of  **29**
Galeazzi fracture  144, 153, 160, 162
Gamekeeper's thumb  178
Gangrene  360–362
    dry  361
    wet  361
Gas gangrene  361
Genu valgum  **23**
Genu varum  **23**
Gerber lift off test  **96**
Gillick competence  9
Glenohumeral joint  87, 90
Glenoid  *88,* 90
Golfer's elbow  *see* Medial epicondylitis
Growth plate fractures  315–319
    anatomy of growth plate  315, *316*
    Salter–Harris classification  317,
        **317**, *317*
    Salter–Harris type II fracture of distal
        tibia  317, *318*

**H**

Haematoma  4
Hallux rigidus  **23**
Hallux valgus  **23**
Hamate fractures  186
Hammertoes  **23**
Hand  *see* Wrist and hand
Hawkins–Kennedy test  **96**
Healing, fracture  4
    and complications  5–6
    stages of  4–5
Heberden's nodes  **22**
Heterotopic ossification  133
High-stepping gait  **29**

Hill–Sachs lesion 108
Hindfoot valgus **23**
Hindfoot varus **23**
Hip 187, 188
  dislocations 193–197
  examination 190–193
  femoral head fractures 218
  femoral shaft fractures 209–212
  femoral triangle *192*
  innervation 189, *191, 192, 193*
  joint anatomy 188, *190*
  movements *194*
  neck of femur fractures 197–209
  osteoarthritis 214–217
  Paget's disease of bone 217–218
  pain 187–188
  periprosthetic fractures 212–214
  prosthetic joint infection 218–219
  radiograph *189*
  surface anatomy 189, *189*
  vascular supply 188–189, *190*
Hip dislocation 193–197
  CT scan in 196
  and fracture of femoral head/neck
    194, *195*
  hip replacement and 194
  posterior 195
  radiographs in 196
Hip spica cast 336, *337*
Histamine test 123
History taking 11, **12**, 14
  age 14, **15**, **16**
  drug history 19
  family history 20
  history of presenting complaint
    18–19
  medical and surgical history 19
  occupation 16–17
  presenting complaint 17–18
  sex 16
  social history 20
  systems review 20
Horner's syndrome 122
Human bite injuries 371–372
Humeral shaft fractures 118–121
  anterioposterior radiograph 119,
    *119*

immobilisation methods 120
open reduction and internal fixation
    120–121
Humerus 87, *88*

**I**

Imaging studies 37–41
  computerised tomography 38–39
  magnetic resonance imaging 40,
    41
  radiography 37–38
  ultrasound 41
Implied consent 6
Infections 355–356
  abscesses 365–366
  bite injuries 371–372
  causative organisms 355
  cellulitis 364–365
  foreign bodies in tissues 369–371
  gangrene 360–362
  necrotising fasciitis 362–363
  neuropathic arthopathy 372–374
  osteomyelitis 358–360
  postoperative wound infections
    363–364
  septic arthritis 356–358
  ulcers 367–369
Informed consent 7
Infraspinatus 90, *91*
Internal iliac artery 222
Intervertebral discs 58–59

**J**

Jobe relocation test **96**
Joint aspiration 41–42, *42*
  diagnostic aspiration 41–42
  prosthetic joint and 43
  therapeutic aspiration 42
Joint crepitus 26
Joint effusion 25
Joint examination 28–32
  feel 31–32
  look 29–31
  move 32
Joint posture 24
Joint stiffness 12–13, 18
  after injury 13, **13**

Joint swelling 11, 18, 27
Jones fractures 304 *see also* Metatarsal fractures

**K**

Kanavel signs 182
Klumpke's palsy 122
Knee 239–241
    ACL rupture 239–240
    anterior view *241*
    bones and articulations 240
    dislocation 267–269
    distal femoral fractures 259–261, *260*
    examination 246–247, *247, 248*
    injuries 239
    innervation 245
    lateral view *243*
    ligaments 243, *244*
    medial view *242*
    osteoarthritis 239, 265–267, *267*
    patella 241–242
    patella dislocations 252–253
    patella fractures 248–251, *249, 250, 251*
    Pellegrini–Stieda lesion 265, *266*
    quadriceps 242, *244*
    soft tissue injuries 263–265
    surface anatomy 246
    tendon injuries 261–263
    tibial plateau fractures 253–257, **256**, *257, 258*
    tibial shaft fractures 257–259
    vascular supply 245, *245*
Knee aspiration 41, *42*
Knee brace 250
Kyphosis 30, 57

**L**

Lachman's test **33**, *248*
Lasègue's sign 56
Lateral epicondylitis 126, 145–146
Leg length, equalisation of 53
Ligaments
    elbow *127*, 127–128
    foot and ankle 272, *273, 274, 275*
    knee 243, *244*
    spine 59, *59*
    wrist and hand 148, *148, 149, 152*
Limb ischaemia 26
Limbs, measurement of 32, 34–35
    arm span 34–35
    calf and thigh circumference 34
    true and apparent leg lengths 34, *35*
Lisfranc injuries 300–302
    anteroposterior radiograph 300, *301*
    CT scan 301
    oblique radiograph 300–301, *302, 303*
Lister's tubercle 168
Living will 9
Lordosis *30*, 57
Loss of function 13–14, **14**
Lumbosacral plexus 222
Lunate dislocations 166–169
    Gilula's arcs 168, *169*
    Mayfield classification **167**

**M**

Magnetic resonance imaging 40, 41
    advantages/disadvantages 40
    contraindications 41
    principles 40
    terminology 40
Maisonneuve fracture 279 *see also* Ankle fracture
Mallet finger **22**, 180, *180*
Mallet toe **23**
March fractures *see* Stress fractures
Medial epicondylitis 146
Median nerve 128
Medications, use of 45–46
Meniscal tears 263–265
Metacarpal fractures 170–173
    acceptable angulation in 172, **172**
    operative treatment 172
    5th metacarpal neck *170*
Metaphyseal fractures, in children 338
Metatarsal fractures 303–308
    avulsion fracture to 5th metatarsal base 305, *305*
    mechanisms of injury 304, **304**

Ottawa foot rules 307
stress fracture 304, 306
Mid-shaft fractures of forearm 153–156
Mondor's sign 295
Mongolian blue spot 340
Monteggia fracture 144
Motion segment 59 *see also* Spine
Muscle atrophy 13
Muscle relaxants 46
Muscle wasting 24

**N**
Nail bed
anatomy of *184*
injuries 183–185
Navicular fractures *310,* 310–311
Neck movements 66, *67*
Neck of femur fractures *see* Proximal femoral fractures
Necrotising fasciitis 362–363, **363**
Needle electromyelography 44
Neer's sign **96**
Nerve conduction studies 44
Neurogenic shock 83
Neuropathic arthopathy 372–374, 373
Neuropraxia **14**
Neurotmesis **14**
Neurovascular status, examination of 36
Nursemaid's elbow *see* Radial head subluxation

**O**
Oculosympathetic palsy 122
Odontoid peg, fractures of 75, *76, 77*
Olecranon *127,* 128
bursitis 145
fractures 137–139, *138, 139*
Open fractures 1–2, 346–349
fracture patterns in 346
Gustilo–Anderson classification 347, **347**
surgical management 348–349
Osteitis deformans *see* Paget's disease of bone
Osteoarthritis, hip 214–217
anteroposterior radiograph 215, *216*

arthroplasty 216
primary 215
secondary 215
Osteoarthritis, knee 239, 265–267
anteroposterior radiograph 266, *267*
conservative management 266
joint replacement 267
Osteogenesis imperfecta 341–342
Osteomyelitis 46, 358–360
causative organism 358
radiographs in 359, *359*
sequestrum 358
Osteotomy 51

**P**
Paediatric orthopaedics
child and adult bones, differences between **313**
condylar fractures 322–327, *323, 324,* **325,** *326*
examination 315
femoral shaft fractures 335–338, **337,** *337*
growth plate fractures 315–319, *316,* **317,** *317, 318*
non-accidental injury 339–341
osteogenesis imperfecta 341–342
Perthes' disease 333–334, *334*
principles of treatment 313
radial head and neck fractures 327–329, *328, 329*
radial head subluxation 329–330
slipped upper femoral epiphysis 330–332, *332*
supracondylar humeral fractures 319–322, *320,* **321,** *321, 322*
tibial fractures 338–339
transient synovitis 313–315, 334–335
Paget's disease of bone 217–218
Pain 11, 17–18
fracture 17
scale of severity of *17*
SOCRATES mnemonic 17
Painful arc test **96**
Paronychia 185

Parsonage–Turner syndrome 121
Passive range of movement 32
Patella 241–242
  bipartite 250, *251*
  dislocations 252–253
  fractures 248–251, *249, 250, 251*
  tension band wiring of 250, *251*
Patellar tap test, for knee effusion 246, *247*
Patellar tendon injuries 261–263, *262*
Patellectomy 250
Pellegrini–Stieda lesion 265, *266*
Pelvic binder 227
Pelvic fracture 221–222, 226–232
  anterior posterior compression (APC) 228, *230*
  lateral compression (LC) 228, *230*
  open reduction and internal fixation 231, *232*
  radiographs in 227, 228
  stable 226
  unstable 226
  vertical shear (VS) 228, *230*
  Young–Burgess classification 228, **229**
Pelvis 221
  anatomy 222–224, *223, 224*
  examination 225
Perilunate dislocations 166–169
  anteroposterior radiograph *166*
  lateral radiograph *167*
Peripheral nerve injury, Seddon classification of **14**
Periprosthetic fractures 212–214
  at stress risers 213
  Vancouver classification 212, *213*
Perthes' disease 333–334, *334*
Pes cavus **23**
Pes planus **23**
Phalangeal fractures 173–176, *174*, 308–310
  classification of 173
  radiographs in 173–174, *174*
  surgical management 175, *175*
Phalen's test **33**
Physiotherapy 45

Pilon fracture 285–288
  anteroposterior radiograph *286*
  distal tibia and 285, *286*
  external fixator application *286*, 288
  non-union 288
Pisiform fractures 186
Plantar fasciitis 311
Plaster of Paris 50
Popeye deformity 123
Popliteal artery, injury to 268
Posterior talofibular ligament 272
Prosthetic joint infection 218–219
Proximal femoral fractures 197–209
  anteroposterior radiograph 199, *200, 201*
  classification 197
  displaced fractures *206*, 206–207, *207*
  fall history 199
  intertrochanteric fractures 207, *208*
  intracapsular fractures 203, **204**, *204*, **205**, *205, 206, 207*
  minimally displaced fractures 205
  risk factors 198
  subtrochanteric fractures 207–209, *208,* **209**
  surgical management 201–203, *202–203*
Proximal humeral fractures 114–118
  anatomy related to 115, *115*
  conservative management 116
  displaced fracture radiograph *117*
  in elderly patients 116
  hemiarthroplasty 116, *118*
  Neer classification 115
  neurovascular anatomy 115, *116*
  open reduction and internal fixation 116, *117*
Pubic rami fractures 231, *231*
Pulled elbow *see* Radial head subluxation

**Q**
Quadriceps 242, *244*
Quadriceps gait **29**
Quadriceps tendon injuries 261–263

**R**

Radial head and neck fractures 141–144, *143*
    anteroposterior radiograph 142, *143*
    associated injuries 142
    in children 327–329, *328, 329*
    Mason classification 142
    radioulnar joint, injury patterns of 142, *143*
Radial head subluxation 329–330
Radial nerve 128
Radiocapitellar line 328
Radiography 37–38
    advantages/disadvantages 38
    principles 37–38
    rule of twos 38
    terminology 38
Rashes 25
Restricted range of motion 27
Rolando fracture 176, *177*
Rotation 3
Rotator cuff 90–91, *91*, 112
    injuries 111–114, *112*

**S**

Sacral fractures 236–238
    CT scan 237, *238*
    radiographs in 237
Saphenous nerve 273, **277**
Scaphoid fractures 162–165, *163, 164*
    scaphoid views 164, *165*
Scapula 87, *89*
    fractures 104–106, *105*
    Y view *105*
Scarf test **33**, **96**
Scars 24
Scissor gait **29**
Scoliosis **22**, *30*
Segond fracture 263, *265*
Septic arthritis 356–358
    causative organisms 357
    Kocher's criteria **357**
Shenton's lines 196
Short leg gait **29**
Shoulder 85, 87
    acromioclavicular joint injuries 102–103

    articulations 90, *91*
    biceps tendon injuries 123–124
    bones 87, *88, 89*
    brachial plexus injuries 121–123
    clavicular fractures 97, 99–102
    dislocations 85–87, 106–111
    examination **96**, 96–97, *98*
    humeral shaft fractures 118–121
    movements *98*
    proximal humeral fractures 114–118
    rotator cuff 90–91, *91*
    rotator cuff injuries 111–114
    scapular fractures 104–106
    surface anatomy 93, *94, 95*
    vascular supply and innervation 91–93, *92*, **93**, *93*
Shoulder dislocations 85–87, 106–111
    anterior dislocations 107–109, *108*
    apprehension test 107
    conservative management 109–111
    inferior dislocation 106
    open procedure 111
    posterior dislocation 106, 109, *109, 110*
    right *107*
    Y view radiographs 108
Signs, in orthopaedic examination 22
    asymmetry 24
    bruising 25
    colour 25
    crepitus 26
    deformities 22, **22–23**
    fixed flexion 26–27
    heat/warmth in joint 27
    joint posture 24
    muscle wasting or weakness 24
    rashes 25
    restricted range of motion 27
    scars 24
    swelling 25, 27
    tenderness 22
    wounds 26
Simmonds' test *see* Calf squeeze test
Skier's thumb 178
Slipped upper femoral epiphysis 330–332, *332*
    frog-leg view of pelvis *332*

operative management 331, *332*
Trethowan's sign *332*
Smith fracture **156**
Social history 20
Speed's test **96**
Spinal anomolies 28, *30*
Spinal cord 59–60, *59–63, 61, 62*
    grey matter 59–60, *61*
    injuries 78–80
    levels of 60, *62*
    meninges 60
    sensory and motor tracts 60–63, *61*
    vascular supply 63
    white matter 60
Spinal fractures 70–71
    burst fractures *72, 72, 73*
    Chance fracture 72–73
    dislocation 73
    wedge fracture 71, *71*
Spinal metastases 80–83
    MRI scan 81, *82*
    pathological wedge fracture 80, *81*
    radiography 80, *81, 82*
    radiotherapy 83–84
    surgical management 84
    winking owl sign of pedicle loss
        due to *82*
Spinal shock 66, 83
Spine 55, 56
    anterior column 57
    cross-section of *58*
    examination 63–64, 66, *67, 68*
    intervertebral discs 58–59
    ligaments 59, *59*
    middle column 58
    movements *68*
    posterior column 58
    regions 56–57, *57*
    spinal cord 59–63, *61, 62*
    surface anatomy 63, *64, 65*
    vertebrae 56, 58, *58*
Stiff hip gait **29**
Stiff knee gait **29**
Straight leg raise test 56
Stress fractures 304, 306 *see also*
    Metatarsal fractures

Subscapularis 90, *91*
Subungual haematomas 184, 309
Superficial peroneal nerve 273, *276,*
    **277,** *277*
Supracondylar fractures 134–136
    CT scan 135, *135*
    plate fixation 136, *136*
    radiographs 135
Supracondylar humeral fractures
    319–322
    Gartland classification 320, **321,** *321*
    Kirschner wires for stabilisation
        322, *322*
    type I fractures 320
    type II fractures 322
    type III fractures 322
Suprapatellar bursa 241
Supraspinatus 90, *91*
Sural nerve 273, *276,* **277,** *277*
Swan neck deformity **23**

T
Talus fractures 291–294
    and avascular necrosis 293–294
    Hawkins classification 292, **292,** *293*
    Hawkins' sign 293, *293*
    lateral process fractures 294, *294*
    radiographs in *292, 293*
Tendon injuries, of hand 178–182, *181*
    extensor tendon injuries 178
    splinting 181
    tendon reconstruction 181
    zones of flexor tendon injury 178,
        *181*
Tendon surgeries 53
Tennis elbow *see* Lateral epicondylitis
Tension band wiring 139
Teres minor 90, *91*
Terrible triad fracture 133
Thomas splint 50–51
Thomas's test **33**
Thompson's test *see* Calf squeeze test
Tibial fractures, in children 338–339
Tibial nerve 273, *276,* **277,** *277*
Tibial plateau fractures 253–257, *257, 258*
    CT scan in 255

and meniscal injuries 255
plate fixation *258*
Schatzker classification 255, **256**
Schatzker type II fracture *257, 258*
Tibial shaft fractures 257–259
Toddler's fracture 339
Torticollis **22**
Transient synovitis 313–315, 334–335
Translation 3
Trauma 18, 343–345
    assessment and management 35
    compartment syndrome 349–352,
        *350*
    open fractures 346–349
    primary survey (ABCDE approach)
        345–346
    vascular injuries 352–354, *354*
Trendelenburg gait **29**
Trendelenburg's test **33**
Triquetral fractures 185–186
Tumour excision 53–54

**U**
Ulcers 367–369, *368*
    in bed-bound patients 369
    in diabetic patients 368
    in vascular patients 368
Ulnar deviation of fingers **23**
Ulnar nerve 128
Ultrasound 41

**V**
Vascular injuries 352–354, *354*
Vertebrae 56, 58, *58, 64*
Volkmann's ischaemic contracture 319

**W**
Wedge fracture, of lumbar vertebrae
    71, *71*

Winging of scapula **22**
Wound infections, postoperative
    363–364
Wounds 26
Wrist and hand 147
    base-of-thumb fractures 176–178,
        *177*
    bones and ligaments of 148, *148,
        149, 152*
    distal radioulnar joint injuries
        160–162, *161*
    distal radius fractures 147–148, **156**,
        156–160, *157, 158, 159*
    examination 151, *153*
    flexor tendon sheath infection
        182–183
    hamate fractures 186
    hand movements *154*
    innervation 150, *150*
    lunate and perilunate dislocations
        *166,* 166–169, **167**, *167, 169*
    metacarpal fractures *170,* 170–173,
        **172**
    mid-shaft fractures of forearm
        153–156
    nail bed injuries 183–185, *184*
    paronychia 185
    phalangeal fractures 173–176,
        *174, 175*
    pisiform fractures 186
    prayer sign *155*
    scaphoid fractures 162–165, *163,
        165*
    surface anatomy *149,* 151, *152*
    tendon injuries 178–182, *181*
    thumb movements *155*
    triquetral fractures 185–186
    vascular supply 150
    wrist movements *153*